Today's
Herbal Health
for
Women

Today's Herbal Health for Women

Louise Tenney, M.H., and Deborah Lee

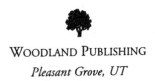

WOODLAND PUBLISHING

Pleasant Grove, UT

The information in this book is for educational purposes only and is not recommended as a means of diagnosing or treating an illness. All matters concerning physical and mental health should be supervised by a health practitioner knowledgeable in treating that particular condition. Neither the publisher nor author directly or indirectly dispense medical advice, nor do they prescribe any remedies or assume any responsibility for those who choose to treat themselves.

Table of Contents

INTRODUCTION   7
SECTION 1: THE DIGESTIVE SYSTEM   9
     Anorexia Nervosa   11
     Gallbladder Problems   13
     Hiatal Hernia   16
     Indigestion   19
     Leaky Gut Syndrome   21
     Ulcers   25
SECTION 2: THE INTESTINAL SYSTEM   31
     Autointoxication   32
     Constipation/Toxic Buildup   36
     Crohn's Disease   44
     Diverticulitis   47
     Irritable Bowel Syndrome   50
SECTION 3: THE URINARY SYSTEM   53
     Bladder and Kidney Infections   54
SECTION 4: THE RESPIRATORY SYSTEM   61
     Respiratory Diseases   62
     Colds, Flu, Fever and Coughs   65
SECTION 5: THE CIRCULATORY AND LYMPHATIC SYSTEMS   73
     Anemia   75
     Bruising   77
     Arteriosclerosis and High Blood Pressure   79
     Varicose Veins and Hemorrhoids   92
SECTION 6: THE GLANDULAR SYSTEM   87
     Glandular Function   89
     Premenstrual Syndrome (PMS)   91
     Cysts and Tumors   95
     Diabetes   99
     Hypoglycemia   103
     Hypothyroidism   107
     Obesity   110
     Cellulite   116

SECTION 7: THE IMMUNE SYSTEM 119
Cancer 121
Allergies 125
Candida (Candidiasis) 130
Epstein Barr and Chronic Fatigue Syndrome 134
Lupus 136
SECTION 8: THE NERVOUS SYSTEM 141
Addictions 142
Anxiety, Panic Attacks and Phobias 147
Chemical Imbalance 151
Depression 155
Autointoxication 158
Insomnia 160
Menniere's Syndrome (Tinnitus) 164
Migraine Headaches 169
SECTION 9: THE STRUCTURAL SYSTEM 173
Arthritis 174
Muscle Disorders 179
Fibromyalgia and Fibrocitis 179
Carpal Tunnel Syndrome 183
Osteoporosis 186
SECTION 10: THE INTEGUMENTARY SYSTEM 191
Hair, Fingernails and Skin Disorders 192
SECTION 11: SPECIAL INTERESTS 197
Herbs Especially for Women 197
Toxic Shock Syndrome 204
Silicone Breast Implants 207
Estrogen 209
Endometriosis 213
"Good" and "Bad" Fats 215
Cholesterol — A Good Thing 219
Menopause 220
Pregnancy 224
Fertility 227
Miscellaneous Issues 231
BIBLIOGRAPHY AND RECOMMENDED READING 237
INDEX 243

Introduction

How can a woman deal with all the problems associated with puberty, pregnancy and menopause? Each phase of a woman's life can be fulfilling if she understands how the body functions and the importance of proper nutrition.

Herbs contain many substances that will clean, balance and build health. They contain minerals, vitamins, oils, enzymes and many other nutrients in their natural and most usable state. They provide materials for the body to correct imbalances and create harmony within the body. Herbs are part of a natural plan designed to keep all living creatures on our planet in optimum health. When used with care, they cause no harmful effects. Herbs provide nutrients in such a way that the body takes what it needs and eliminates what is not utilized.

The wisdom of our ancestors is being validated today — herbs are plants that people have used for thousands of years. Our ancestors passed their knowledge down through the ages and developed numerous remedies that proved effective for their health challenges. Modern researchers have proven that herbs are effective because they contain the necessary nutrients to help the body heal itself.

Herbs are used as preventive medicine, as well as for healing. They are compatible with the body, providing nourishment and vitality to the female organs. The purpose of herbs is to help the woman obtain harmony, health and happiness in every phase of her life.

white blood cells are part of the immune system, and always increase in number when there is a need to eliminate hostile invaders. This would indicate that a diet comprising primarily of cooked food can initiate the beginnings of inflammation or disease. Cooked food places an added burden on the immune system, as well as contributes to digestive disturbances. It is no wonder we have so many auto-immune diseases plaguing us today. Eating raw food does not increase white cell response. Eating raw vegetables before cooked food prevents the appearance of extra white cells. This was discovered by a famous Swiss nutritionist, Dr. Bircher-Benner. A salad with endive or watercress is very beneficial for digestion and will heal and repair the stomach.

Proper digestion depends on a healthy appetite. A healthy appetite depends on live, nourishing food, and the images it creates in our minds. The smell and taste of food helps prepare the body for its digestion. Digestion begins with sensations of hunger and starts the saliva glands working. Saliva is important for digesting carbohydrates. Improper digestion of carbohydrates can cause autointoxication and gas in the large intestine.

The small intestine is vital to the digestion and absorption of the food we eat. The small intestine changes the food into useable material like glucose, fatty acids and amino acids. The type of food we eat determines the nutrients we will receive in our bloodstream. Digestion is completed by enzymes secreted in the intestinal juices of the small intestine. Disruption, disease or digestive problems interfere with the small intestine's main job of absorbing nutrients. If the small intestine is healthy, these nutrients move at a normal rate and are absorbed and assimilated. The waste material is then carried on to the large intestine. If there is a thick coating of mucus on the intestinal walls, or if the intestines are irritated and move nutrients too quickly, the body will receive very little nourishment. If the proteins are not properly digested, they ferment into poisons such as phenol, indol and skatol. These poisons are then absorbed into the bloodstream and cause a breakdown in the system. Emotional stress plays a major role in stomach digestive disorders. The stomach is a very sensitive organ and nervous problems can slow down or speed up digestion. Under acute stress, the stomach has a tendency to shut off acid production. Chronic stress also causes an excessive excretion of hydrochloric acid, which can cause acid indigestion. This irritation of the mucous membrane lining of the stomach may cause ulcers and hiatal hernias. It is a big mistake to eat while under emotional stress.

Anorexia Nervosa

Anorexia is an eating disorder found mostly among young women who have a fear of getting fat and gaining even a little weight. They try to avoid food altogether. One third of those involved eventually die. It is a more emotionally devastating sickness, a starvation disease.

SYMPTOMS

- broken blood vessels on the face and neck (from vomiting)
- extreme weakness
- depression and lack of self-worth
- erosion of enamel on teeth (vomiting acids)
- dehydration, loss of minerals and fluids
- electrolyte imbalance
- dry skin and hair
- cessation of menstruation
- heart palpitations or low blood pressure

CAUSES

Society is obsessed with thinness, which is exploited on television and in magazines. Perfectionism can be a cause. It is difficult to change an anorexic's mind. A vicious cycle causes a loss of appetite from nutritional deficiencies and vice-versa. Anorexics abandon all responsibility of a healthy body for the strong will to control themselves. A poor relationship with parents can be a cause. It is a very serious disease and can eventually kill a person if they do not turn their life around. Hormonal imbalance is another cause; it can stem from constipation and autointoxication. Lack of minerals can weaken the heart and cause heart failure.

NATURAL TREATMENT

Increasing the appetite may help stimulate the desire to nourish the body. Learning about the body and the importance of nutrition help victims and sufferers to understand the role of food in nourishing the body. Emotions need to be dealt with as well.

If a young girl has the will, she should be able to eat right and gain weight. Nourishing foods include whole grains, almonds and almond milk, vegetables, fruit, sprouts, and homemade vegetable soups. The nerves and the brain need to be nourished so reasoning can be accomplished. You can reason with a person whose brain is fed properly.

DIETARY GUIDELINES

Prepare grain and vegetable soups and make a broth to begin with so it will be easy to eat, digest and assimilate. Use leeks, garlic, and parsley, which are rich in copper and other nutrients. This will provide minerals to stimulate the appetite and prevent weakness and disease in the body. Pure lemon and ginger juice in a glass of water will stimulate the appetite. A fresh juice drink made with carrot, celery, parsley and ginger is rich in minerals, especially zinc. Millet is high in calcium and magnesium and is easy to digest and assimilate.

NUTRITIONAL SUPPLEMENTS

Zinc deficiency contributes to anorexia. When a person is deficient in minerals and vitamins, it can decrease the appetite.

Amino Acid Supplements are essential for maintaining health of the body. They help restore normal function to the metabolic connection of the brain. A healthy mind will be able to solve health problems or obsessive behavior. Extra phenylalanine, thyrosine and methionine will help improve emotional health. Glutamic acid is an important amino acid for the brain. Taking this amino acid increases desire in some to face and admit their problems.

Plant Digestive Enzymes will assure the food eaten is properly digested and assimilated.

Acidophilus is essential for restoring friendly bacteria to the intestines. It also helps in digestion and assimilation of nutrients.

Chlorophyll is beneficial for building the blood and increasing the appetite. It supplies essential nutrients for the body. A liquid vitamin and mineral supplement will be easy to assimilate and digest, and will help restore health faster.

Essential Fatty Acids include the following oils, which can be used in a combination to help restore health to the glandular system: evening primrose, borage, flaxseed, salmon, and black currant.

Kelp is rich in minerals. A combination of kelp, dulse, alfalfa, licorice, dandelion, and yellow dock is rich in nutrients.

Nervine Formulas help in emotional stability. These include: hops, valerian, skullcap, white willow, passion flower and St. John's wort.

Brain Formula, with *Ginkgo biloba,* gotu kola, suma, bee pollen, Siberian ginseng and capsicum will increase circulation to the brain.

Co Q-10 and Germanium will provide oxygen to the blood and brain.

Vitamin B-Complex helps in eliminating toxins from the liver, and improves digestion. It is also important for strengthening the nerves.

Goldenseal improves appetite and normalize digestive juices. It also helps in chronic constipation, gives tone to the digestive system and improves nervous stomach.

Facts at a Glance

• Anorexia can eventually lead to heart failure and death.
• Nutritional deficiencies create a loss of appetite.
• A severe lack of zinc is implicated in anorexia.
• Emotional instability is seen in cases of obsessive behavior.
• Anorexics usually keep their obsessive behavior from everyone else. This creates a loneliness and anti-social feeling.

Gallbladder Problems

About twelve million American women suffer from gallstones, the most common illness associated with the gallbladder. The gallbladder becomes congested when the liver is overburdened with toxins, and the excess goes to the gallbladder which has a limited capacity to store bile. The bile breaks down the fat, which is then absorbed by the small intestine. When too much sediment, cholesterol or inorganic minerals accumulate, the gallbladder becomes congested and inefficient.

Bile in the gallbladder contains bile salts and cholesterol. The cholesterol is necessary to act as a buffer agent, preventing bile acids from eating away at the gallbladder and small intestine. Our bodies need cholesterol, which acts as an antioxidant against free-radical damage.

SYMPTOMS

- pain and tenderness on right side of body
- blocked cystic duct causes inflammation
- fever and jaundice
- back pain
- liver congestion causes sluggishness
- nausea and vomiting

CAUSES

Women seem to be more prone to gallstones than men. One reason for this is that the excess estrogen in the liver can cause an imbalance. A high-fat and -meat diet can lead to gallstones. A low-fiber diet can lead to gallbladder problems. Younger women seem to be more prone when on oral contraceptives.

Those overweight who eat a lot of dairy products and animal fats are more prone to gallstones. Overweight women cannot utilize fat and it will cause liver and gallbladder problems as well as excess weight. Pregnant women who do not eat high-fiber food are also prone to gallstones. A rapid weight change can cause gallstones.

NATURAL TREATMENT

Exercise and maintain a proper weight. Change the diet using more vegetables and grains and less meat. We need cholesterol in our bodies, but we also need more fiber to help balance cholesterol levels. The colon and liver need to be cleaned because a congested colon causes the toxins to circulate in the bloodstream and cause the liver and gallbladder to enlarge and become less effective.

DIETARY GUIDELINES

Change from a high-fat and meat diet to more vegetables, rice and grains, such as millet, buckwheat, whole oats, kamut, wheat, and rye, which will add fiber, vitamins and minerals. Drink plenty of pure water daily.

Juices to help with the gallbladder are a combination of carrot, celery and endive, garlic and ginger. Endive has bitter properties to increase bile; garlic and ginger protect the gallbladder and liver.

NUTRITIONAL SUPPLEMENTS

Lecithin emulsifies fat and is important for the maintenance of soluble bile to prevent gallstones.

L-Carnitine eliminates fat in the blood and around the heart.

Vitamin C with bioflavonoids are necessary for gallbladder health. Vitamin C helps convert cholesterol into bile salts and helps prevent formation of gall stones.

Vitamin E improves circulation and prevents abnormal clotting. It also prevents fats from becoming rancid.

B-complex Vitamins are involved in the breakdown of carbohydrates, fats and proteins for energy. They help prevent the formation of gallstones and nourish the liver and gallbladder. They improve hormone production from adrenal glands.

Supplements of Vitamins A, D, E and K are essential when gallbladder problems are present.

Blue-green Algae and Chlorophyll nourish the spleen and liver to prevent accumulation of hard bile.

Gallbladder Cleanse — FIRST DAY: No food to be taken, 8:00 am — 1 glass (8 oz.) fresh apple juice, then 2 glasses (16 oz.) fresh apple juice at 10:00 am, 12:00 am, 2:00 pm, 4:00 pm and 6:00 pm. SECOND DAY: Same as first; at bedtime take 4 oz of pure olive oil in 18 oz. of warm pure water with 1 juiced lemon or warm apple juice. Retire and lay on your right side. It should start working in the early morning. The malic acid from the apple juice helps dissolve the stagnant bile and the oil moves the residue.

Facts At A Glance

• Gallbladder problems are common in women.
• Too much fat overstimulates the gallbladder.
• A gallbladder cleanse helps in dissolving and eliminating gallstones.
• A high-fiber diet is beneficial.

Hiatal Hernia

Hiatal hernia is a very common condition that affects over fifty percent of the population of the United States over forty years of age. It occurs when a small portion of the stomach slips through an opening (hiatus) in the diaphragm, forcing the stomach to push into the chest. Leakage of acid in the lower esophagus is the reason for the discomfort, and will cause inflammation and irritation. If it continues, it can cause ulceration, scarring and even blockage of the esophagus.

Symptoms

• belching
• burning sensation
• regurgitation of food causing burning and pain
• intestinal gas
• constipation (can push the stomach upwards)
• nausea and lack of appetite (fear of belching or regurgitation of food)
• discomfort is aggravated when lying down after eating

Causes

A low-fiber diet is one of the main causes of a hiatal hernia. It creates constipation, which in turn causes straining, which may protrude the stomach. Carbonated drinks cause irritation to the stomach and esophagus. Eating the wrong combination of food will cause fermentation and gas which will irritate the stomach.

Lack of hydrochloric acid and digestive enzymes can cause an imbalance in the digestive process. A high-meat and -fat diet as well as cooked food cause enzyme depletion and indigestion.

Eating when under stress causes a tightening of the digestive organs and slows down digestion, putting stress on the adrenal glands.

Overeating, antacid consumption, bad diet, alcohol, and tobacco, too many white flour and white sugar products and lack of minerals can all contribute to a hiatal hernia.

NATURAL TREATMENT

Learn how to combine food properly. Eat smaller meals. Avoid artificial coloring, additives such as MSG and carbonated drinks. Avoid eating meat and sugar at the same meal. (This causes fermentation and creates gas and indigestion.)

A chiropractor or massage therapist can put the hernia back into place. Dr. Theodore A. Baroody, Jr., says in his book *Hiatal Hernia Syndrome,* to simply drink 16 oz. of water and bounce on the heels 12 times. This puts weight in the stomach, and the bouncing will jar it into place.

DIETARY GUIDELINES

Eat fresh salads before meals and chew thoroughly. Add plant digestive enzymes to meals to ensure proper digestion, and so that protein in cells and blood can break down and be eliminated. Eat plenty of steamed vegetables and avoid too much table salt, which will inhibit enzyme utilization.

Eat a high-fiber diet such as brown rice, millet, rye, whole oats, kamut and buckwheat. Use beans, sprouts, and raw almonds. A fresh juice drink made with green cabbage, celery, carrots and fresh ginger is healing. Learn relaxation methods to avoid stress on the body.

Nutritional Supplements

Aloe Vera is healing and will prevent scarring.

Antioxidants, such as Vitamins A, C, E, selenium and zinc will heal and prevent scarring. They will nourish the mucous membranes of the digestive tract and strengthen the immune system.

Essential Fatty Acids (flaxseed, borage, salmon oil, black currant, and evening primrose oil) have a healing effect and nourish the glands.

Licorice Root soothes the digestive tract. It also promotes healing of peptic, gastric and duodenal ulcers, which are sometime involved with hiatal hernias.

Blue-Green Algae and Chlorophyll nourish the digestive tract and promote interferon production for immune protection.

Amino Acid Supplements, such as a free-form, "predigested" amino acids do not need stomach acid for digestion and help the body supply the acid required. Should be used with extra hydrochloric acid and digestive enzymes.

Goldenseal is a bitter tonic and provides healing properties for the digestive tract. It will help expel worms and relieve chronic constipation.

Herbs that help the digestive tract include aloe vera, slippery elm, fenugreek, burdock, cat's claw, ginger, licorice, goldenseal, comfrey, pau d'arco, marshmallow and St. John's wort.

Blood Cleansing Herbs include burdock, watercress, sorrel, slippery elm and turkey rhubarb. They clean the blood and strengthen the immune system.

Colon Cleansing herbs, which include cascara sagrada, barberry, raspberry leaves, lobelia, ginger, rhubarb, goldenseal, fennel, and cayenne, will help clean, heal and rebuild a sluggish colon.

Facts At A Glance

- Hiatal hernia is common in persons over forty.
- A high-fiber diet is important in preventing a hiatal hernia.
- Hydrochloric acid and digestive enzymes are important.
- Carbonated drinks cause irritation in the digestive tract.

Indigestion

The digestive system is responsible for feeding the cells properly and preventing illness. Digestive problems are very common and cause an imbalance in the body. Toxins are allowed to accumulate and cause cell degeneration and oxidation. The immune system is weakened and resistance to disease is decreased. The body becomes sluggish and heavier, the skin becomes blotchy and emotions can become unstable. Many diseases are manifested when improper digestion exists.

The new drugs advertised to prevent heartburn will eventually cause more problems. The stomach needs hydrochloric acid to destroy germs, virus, bacteria, parasites and worms. It is usually the lack of hydrochloric acid that causes heartburn. Some of the drugs are Pepcid®, Axid®, Tagamet® and Zantac®. They used to be prescribed for ulcers, and now can be bought over the counter.

SYMPTOMS

- belching
- full and uncomfortable feeling after eating
- gas
- heartburn
- pain in stomach
- headaches
- nausea

CAUSES

The main causes of indigestion are overeating, constipation, wrong combinations of food, too much caffeine, alcohol, tobacco, sweets, white flour products and over-cooked food. Too much meat and dairy products are high in fat which is very hard on digestion. Stress is also involved. Stomach problems may also be caused by a refusal to accept life's problems, and may indicate a hidden fear of life, tension and nervous disorders. An imbalance in the body contributes to digestive problems.

Lack of hydrochloric acid and enzymes can also contribute to digestive problems. *Candida* overgrowth can cause indigestion. Colon and liver congestion can cause ulcers, indigestion and stomach inflammation. Other causes of indigestion may be allergies, hiatal hernia, gallbladder problems, stress, ulcers or heart problems.

NATURAL TREATMENT

Avoid lying down after eating. Walking will help stimulate better digestion. Avoid antacids; they only treat the symptoms. Find the cause and treat accordingly. When under stress, don't eat. Wait for a more calming atmosphere; a relaxed eating environment improves digestion.

DIETARY GUIDELINES

Nourish the digestive tract with fresh juices made with green cabbage, celery, carrots and ginger. Millet is very easy to digest and is healing. Vegetable broths are rich in minerals — especially potassium, which is important for the digestive tract. Herbal teas using chamomile, licorice, comfrey, fenugreek, goldenseal and aloe vera are soothing.

Eat smaller meals and chew the food very well so the digestive enzymes in the saliva can be stimulated. Predigested amino acids will help stimulate enzyme activity in the stomach.

Cook grains in the thermos overnight and chew them thoroughly. They contain live enzymes and are rich in minerals and vitamins.

A high-fiber diet is necessary to restore health to the digestive tract. Fresh papaya and pineapple help supply digestive enzymes. Use frozen juices if you cannot get the tree-ripened fruit; they are better than the canned juices. Blood, liver and colon herbal formulas will help clean and heal the digestive tract.

NUTRITIONAL SUPPLEMENTS

Acidophilus protects against overgrowth of bad bacteria, and also helps in the digestion of food.

Blue-green Algae helps in the digestion in food while supplying essential vitamins and minerals.

Antioxidants help in preventing free-radical damage. Examples are vitamin A, vitamin C with bioflavonoids, vitamin E, minerals such as selenium and zinc, and grape seed extract.

B-complex Vitamins are essential for a healthy digestive tract. They are involved in eliminating toxins from the liver.

Amino Acids (predigested) are healing for the digestive tract and stimulate enzyme activity.

Digestive Enzymes are essential for healing and restoring health to the digestive tract, organs and cells of the body. They help break up and eliminate congested protein in the blood, cells and organs.

Minerals are essential for relieving indigestion, especially calcium, magnesium and zinc. Potassium is also excellent for healing.

Herbs that soothe the stomach include catnip, chamomile, anise seeds, ginger, aloe vera, licorice and peppermint.

FACTS AT A GLANCE

• Indigestion is a very common problem.
• Diseases are manifested when digestion is a problem.
• Lack of hydrochloric acid and enzymes can cause indigestion.
• Digestive aids on the market can only create more problems.

Leaky Gut Syndrome

A syndrome is a group of signs and symptoms that collectively characterize or indicate particular diseases or abnormal conditions. One disease, like arthritis, may have a certain number of symptoms, but if another symptom occurs that the medical profession doesn't connect with arthritis, they give it another name, such as joint disease, soft tissue disorders, ankylosing spondylitis, and connective tissue disorders such as lupus or gout, and the list goes on.

Dr. Sherry A. Rogers, M.D., explains leaky gut syndrome: "The leaky gut syndrome is a poorly recognized, but extremely common problem that is seldom tested for. It represents a hyperpermeable intestinal lining. In other words, large spaces develop between the cells of the gut wall and bacteria, toxins and foods leak in" (*Let's Live,* April 1995, 34-35). The body lacks enzymes to help digest the protein in our blood and cells. We can only get enzymes from raw food and digestive enzyme supplements. When we eat cooked food, the T cells come to the stomach, as they see this as foreign matter. But when we eat raw food this does not happen. The T cells are the protection of the immune system, and when we continually overstimulate our protective system, we eventually wear it out. This may be one reason why we have so many autoimmune diseases. A large part of the population of the United States chronically suffer from one or more of these disorders. As long as we play games with the immune system and interfere with the body's only protection, we will see more and more unusual autoimmune diseases.

The widespread use of vaccinations and antibiotics is considered one of the main causes of immune system disorders. Now we are seeing prescribed drugs for ulcers put on the market to prevent acid indigestion. Axid®, Zantac® and Pepcid® can now be purchased over the counter. They are advertised to take before you eat to prevent indigestion. If these are used, we are going to see more diseases develop. A hyperacidic stomach usually means you are lacking hydrochloric acid or Candida is present in the stomach. Hydrochloric acid is essential to digest protein, for the assimilation of minerals, and to destroy worms, parasites, germs, bacteria and viruses.

SYMPTOMS

- fatigue (one of the first signs of an autoimmune disease)
- aches and pains
- colds and flu are common
- frequent infections
- chronic low-grade fever
- fungal diseases (yeast, *Candida,* fungi)
- nausea, vomiting, pain after eating

Causes

The main cause of leaky gut syndrome is a bad diet, void of enzymes. The glands are overworked, trying to provide the enzymes we are not obtaining in our diet. When we eat cooked food we over-stimulate the immune system and wear it out, and it loses the ability to protect us. Therefore, we leave the body vulnerable for any disease that comes along. The wide use of drugs and vaccinations further weaken our bodies and invite germs and viruses to thrive.

The chemicals, heavy metals, pesticides and herbicides in our food, air and water further weaken our body and injure the digestive system.

Cell membranes are also weakened when we do not treat colds, flu, and all acute diseases naturally and let them run their course. When we treat them with antibiotics, aspirin, antihistamines, and flu and cold drugs, this only suppresses the toxins that are trying to be eliminated from the body. If we treat them naturally, stop eating, only drink citrus juices, and take herbs and broths, the body will heal itself. The toxins, proteins, and viruses will not build up in the blood and cells.

Natural Treatment

The intestinal tract can be healed by adding more raw food to the diet, especially fresh vegetable juices. Fasting on vegetable juices will help repair and provide enzymes for a healthy body. They are rich in enzymes and will help to build up the reserve in our glands. If sixty to seventy percent of our diet consists of raw foods, there is a chance we can reverse bodily degeneration and provide more energy and vitality.

Cleansing the digestive tract and the colon will help assure that the body is digesting and assimilating the necessary nutrients for healing and restoring proper function. We need to make certain that we are eliminating after every meal. A low-fiber diet consisting mostly of cooked food, white flour, sugar products, and greasy food will encrust the colon and cause autointoxication. This causes chronic diseases. It has taken years to build up, so be patient in eliminating these toxins. Use a fiber formula, blood cleanser, and lower bowel formula to clean out the toxins.

DIETARY GUIDELINES

Beneficial juices are a combination of carrot, celery, endive and fresh ginger, or carrot, parsley, cabbage and garlic, or ginger, parsley, garlic, carrots and celery. Fasting on these juices two to three days a week will speed healing of the digestive tract.

Eat thermos-cooked grains. They are rich in enzymes, vitamins, minerals and protein, which will heal the digestive tract. This is a slow way to cook, and prevents destruction of vital enzymes.

Drink plenty of liquids, especially pure water, electrolyte drinks (without sugar, if possible), and fruit juices diluted with pure water. Almond milk drinks are rich in calcium, magnesium and protein. Use almond milk to make fruit drinks.

Millet, buckwheat and basmati brown rice can be used in breakfast meals. These are easy to digest and nourishing. Add plenty of steamed vegetables, yams and avocados. Eat broths made with grains and vegetables. These are also healing and nourishing.

NUTRITIONAL SUPPLEMENTS

Acidophilus destroys putrefactive bacteria in the intestinal tract. Putrefactive bacteria liberates histamine, a toxic substance that is the result of undigested protein. Vitamin K and B-vitamins can be synthesized in the small intestine by using acidophilus.

Plant Digestive Enzymes will help digest food, and when taken between meals will help break up the protein in the blood and cells, so the body can eliminate the toxins.

Vitamin A (beta-carotene) is vital for tissue repair.

B-complex Vitamins are essential for intestinal health. They help prevent depression, fatigue, sugar cravings, bloating and weight fluctuation. They also help eliminate the "bad estrogen" from the liver.

Vitamin C with bioflavonoids is necessary for the adrenal and thyroid gland to supply hormones. It is vital for collagen health, help in absorption of calcium, and is necessary for a healthy digestive tract.

Vitamins A, C, E, Selenium and Zinc are antioxidants. They protect the cells from damage, especially the lungs and immune system.

Minerals are essential for a healthy digestive tract. Calcium and magnesium improve nerve health, regulate heartbeat, and strengthen muscles. Zinc speeds healing. Minerals are essential to for enzymes to work in the body.

Essential Fatty Acids are needed for healthy glands. They help regulate hormones. Examples include flaxseed oil, salmon, evening primrose, borage, and black currant oils.

Blue-green Algae and Chlorophyll cleanse and heal the digestive tract and clean the blood.

Aloe Vera Juice heals and repairs tissue in the digestive tract.

Herbs valuable to the health of the digestive tract include cat's claw, grape seed extract, pau d'arco, licorice, goldenseal, slippery elm, comfrey, and horsetail.

FACTS AT A GLANCE

- Leaky gut syndrome is more common than we realize.
- Bad diet with low fiber and too much cooked food has created this syndrome.
- Digestive enzymes are necessary for healing a leaky gut syndrome, as well as preventing autoimmune diseases. Use live food as well as plant digestive enzyme supplements.
- Supplements will speed healing of the digestive tract.
- Colon cleaning is essential for eliminating toxins and healing and restoring health to the entire digestive tract.

Ulcers

There is a widespread belief among doctors that ulcers are caused by a spiral-shaped virus called *Helicobactes pylori* (HP). It is no wonder that viruses and bacteria form in the intestinal tract when antacids are widely prescribed. Any time the hydrochloric acid is decreased, viruses, parasites and worms thrive in the stomach and other parts of the intestinal system. *H. pylori* is found in a large number of patients suffering from stomach and duodenal ulcers.

We believe the germs come when toxins are already in the body. Then when drugs, such as Zantac® and Tagamet®, are prescribed to neutralize or suppress stomach acid, the germs, worms, and viruses can thrive.

These drugs are very popular. They control the ulcers but when the drugs are stopped the ulcers often come back. As many as 60 to 90 percent of ulcer suffers have a relapse. Now these are advertised as over-the-counter antacids. We are going to see more autoimmune disease, stomach problems, worms and parasites invading the body. The most common ulcers are found in the duodenum and in the lower part of the stomach.

In the past, the medical field would recommend a low-fiber diet that included milk. The milk does neutralize acid, but in the long run causes the stomach to secrete more acid. Lack of fiber is seen as another cause of ulcers.

SYMPTOMS

- gnawing pain in the abdomen, mostly when stomach is empty
- heartburn
- nausea
- bleeding
- vomiting

CAUSES

Stress can play a major role in ulcers, but there has to be more to cause the stomach to form sores, like autointoxication and constipation. When the lower colon is clogged and delays the passage of food from the stomach, fermentation and acid conditions will irritate the stomach wall. We are also wearing out our digestive system by continually eating cooked food. The glands are continually producing enzymes to help in the digestion process and become overworked. The pancreas swells when we eat too much cooked food. Mucus is formed every time we eat cooked food and this leaves our stomach vulnerable to all kinds of germs, viruses and toxins.

NATURAL TREATMENT

Eat only when hungry and not while under stress. When the body is under stress it secretes stomach acid. This depletes the acid that is really needed to digest food. Learn to treat acute diseases naturally, and eliminate aspirin, and all drugs that suppress the symptoms. Use herbs, vitamins, minerals, juices and mild food.

There are special herbal formulas to clean the stomach, bowels and liver. They will help heal and repair the lining of the stomach. The stomach will heal itself when given the correct nutrients.

Eliminate foods that cause distress to give the stomach a chance to heal. Meat, dairy products, milk and cheese can make an ulcer worse. Stay away from coffee, alcohol, soft drinks, sugar and white flour products. A high-fiber diet will help clean and eliminate toxins.

DIETARY GUIDELINES

Use cabbage, celery and carrot juice often. Cabbage juice has been proven to heal ulcers. You can add ginger juice to the above juices. Millet is easy to digest and nourishing. It is rich in calcium and magnesium and protein. Eat more fruit, steamed vegetables and whole grains. Potato peel broth is healing. Make grain and vegetable soups. Barley helps rebuild the stomach lining. It is rich in B1, B2 and bioflavonoids. Cook slowly in a thermos to retain the enzymes and B-vitamins.

Make a tea from flaxseeds. It will coat and heal the ulcers. Avocados, bananas, yams and cooked carrots are also healing.

Eat more whole grains, such as brown rice, millet, buckwheat, whole oats, kamut, amaranth, quinoa and rye. Grains supply trypophan in the body which converts into seratonin and melatonin in the brain.

The following is a recipe for a very healthy enzyme drink, sometimes referred to as "rejuvelac." This drink is a predigested food. The proteins are broken down into amino acids and the carbohydrates into simple sugars. These nutrients are readily assimilated by the body, with little energy going for digestion. To make this drink, you will need:

1 cup wheat berries (organic, soft pastry wheat)
3 cups pure water
1 quart jar with a wide mouth

Be sure to use untreated wheat berries. Wash the wheat and remove any old or bad ones. Use your hands to scrub, and let the bad ones float to the top so they can be discarded. Soak the wheat berries for 48 hours. After 48 hours, pour off the rejuvelac, which is ready to use. It will keep for several days without refrigeration. Good rejuvelac has a pleasant odor and tastes somewhat sour and lemony taste. Keep in a dark and warm place while soaking. Seventy degrees farenheit is the ideal temperature for soaking. Pour two more cups of pure water into the jar of wheat berries. Let this ferment for 24 hours before pouring off. It can be repeated again for 24 more hours. The wheat berries can be soaked a total of three times.

NUTRITIONAL SUPPLEMENTS

Food Enzymes are essential to clean and repair the stomach. Use them with meals and between meals for healing.

Licorice (*Glycyrrhiza glabra*) has been shown to have anti-ulcer properties without side effects. It seems to stimulate growth and regenerate stomach and intestinal cells.

Essential Fatty Acids include flaxseed oil, borage, evening primrose, salmon, and black currant oils. They will coat and heal the ulcers. They also feed and nourish the glands.

Aloe Vera juice is healing and will soothe and help in pain.

Capsicum stops bleeding and will heal ulcers.

Goldenseal is healing for ulcers and contains antibiotic and antibacterial properties.

Free-form Amino Acid supplements are essential for healing and repairing tissues.

Fiber supplements will help prevent ulcers and aid in healing the lining of the intestines. High fiber foods can increase bulk in the intestines and eliminate invading bacteria, worms, parasites and germs that accumulate in the intestines.

Guar Gum and Psyllium have mild laxative effects and create bulk to help the body eliminate waste without straining.

Red Raspberry and Chamomile Teas are relaxing and healing for the intestines.

Comfrey, Fenugreek, Burdock, Garlic, Black Walnut, Dandelion, Echinacea, Ginger, Myrrh, Cat's Claw, Pau d'Arco, and Milk Thistle are all healing and cleansing for the intestines.

FACTS AT A GLANCE

• Dietary changes will prevent and heal ulcers.

• Drugs control ulcers, but ulcers often come back when the drugs are stopped.

• Enzymes will help heal and repair the stomach.

• Fasting on juices, especially green cabbage, will help heal ulcers.

Section 2

The Intestinal System

Healing is a matter of time, but it is sometimes also a matter of opportunity.

HIPPOCRATES

The Body's Waste Elimination Station

It is estimated that close to ninety percent of all ailments plaguing humankind begin in a toxic and constipated colon. Poisons from the colon can weaken and stress the heart, can lodge in the joints and cause stiffness and pain, can invade the muscles and cause fatigue and weakness, can enter the brain and cause senility and brain fatigue, and can cause the skin to eliminate in the form of blemishes, psoriasis, liver spots, wrinkles and bumps, and can irritate the lungs and cause asthma, bronchitis and bad breath.

Dr. Henry A. Cotton, in 1932, wrote a paper about the pathology of intestinal toxemia. He had studied the colon's removal from insane patients for years and revealed one or more of the following characteristic changes in the bowel: destruction of the epithelium and mucosa; areas of hemorrhage, pigmentation and ulceration; extreme atrophy of the muscular coats, with the bowel wall thinned in places to a parch-ment-like consistency, resulting in dilated, pouchy areas referred to by Cotton as "segmental blowouts"; marked thickening of the bowel wall due to chronic fibrous tissue growth; after a colectomy or a post-mortem inspection, in every instance showed various types of strepto-cocci and virulent colon bacilli; also diverticulosis.

It is significant to know that the colon is in even worse shape in the majority of people today than it was at the turn of the century. Diets are low in fiber and waste material accumulates because of the glue-like food we ingest daily. The body needs pure water. Inorganic minerals, toxic metals, worms and parasites help create constipation and accu-mulate in the body and produce toxic waste material. When a person eats under stress, it can cause indigestion and constipation. Eating wholesome food on a regular basis, employing proper sleeping habits, and regular exercise will help the intestinal system stay healthy.

Autointoxication

Autointoxication, or intestinal toxemia, is a condition that creates an internal environment where bacteria, germs and viruses can feed, multiply and flourish. Autointoxication, along with leaky gut syn-drome, are the main causes of humankind's illnesses.

A healthy colon is essential in order to heal the body, as well as pre-vent diseases. When there is a delay in the movement of food along the digestive tract, fermentation or putrefaction quickly develops. If this condition remains in the body more than 24 hours, toxins can be reab-sorbed into the bloodstream, and then distributed throughout the body. Every cell, tissue and organ are subsequently bathed with these poisons.

Many years can pass before symptoms of a chronic disease appear. The reason is that the body has provided means of cleansing through the skin, lungs and kidneys. After a while, the defense system breaks down; the mucous membranes become the seat of infection with col-itis and diverticulitis. This allows even a larger amount of poisons to pass into the bloodstream. It causes the liver, thyroid and the kidneys to become overworked and damaged in an effort to remove the toxins from the blood.

We now see the effects of chronic disease manifesting itself. Every organ and function of the body show evidence of damage. The poisons circulating in the blood irritate the walls of the blood vessels and cause hardening of the arteries. The brain and nervous system show signs of depression or irritation, especially if "bad" estrogen is in the blood. The lungs become irritated and bronchitis, pneumonia and bad breath develop. And when the digestive system is irritated we have digestive problems, leaky gut syndrome and ulcers.

SYMPTOMS

- headaches (an imbalance in the liver and colon)
- lower back pain (inflammation of the sciatic nerve)
- depression (toxins can enter the brain)
- fatigue (toxins in the bloodstream)
- aches and pains (toxins in the weakest part of the body)
- skin blemishes (age spots from free radical damage)
- anxiety, and irritability (the nervous system is irritated)
- premenstrual syndrome (hormone imbalance from bad estrogen)
- allergies, arthritis, asthma, irregular heartbeat, ear, nose and throat diseases, toxemia of pregnancy, eye disease, nervous system diseases, senility, and cancer

CAUSES

Constipation is the cause of autointoxication. The main factors are lack of fiber; eating cooked food, which is void of enzymes; eating white flour products, which act like glue in the colon; fried food, which also adheres to the colon; lack of exercise, which weakens the muscle tone of the colon; eating wrong combinations of food, and eating food and drinks which are constipating.

Constipating foods and drinks are cheese, meat, fried food, white sugar products, white flour products, dairy products, carbonated drinks, alcohol and coffee.

Natural Treatment

The body will start healing and cleansing with juice fasting. Wheatgrass juice or a juice drink made from the following are cleansing for the colon: celery, carrot, parsley, endive and green leafy lettuce. Green drinks are cleansing for the colon. Colon cleansing is essential to dissolve the crust on the colon walls. Do juice fasting one or two days a week. Enemas and colonics are very helpful in helping to loosen the crust on the colon walls.

Use lower bowel formulas and herbs that clean the liver, blood and colon. This will help balance the chemistry of the body, and the hormones.

Exercise is essential to strengthen the colon. Sitting exercises, a rowing machine and jumping on a trampoline will help strengthen the colon.

Dietary Guidelines

Add more fiber to the diet to speed the transit time of food through the intestinal tract. Start with a fiber supplement which contains the following: psyllium, guar gum, burdock, rhubarb root, black walnut, red raspberry, pumpkin seed, and other herbs as needed. Increase the use of whole grains, such as brown rice, millet, whole oats, kamut, quinoa, buckwheat, whole wheat and yellow corn meal.

Use raw salads, steamed vegetables, beans, whole wheat bread, sprouts, and fresh fruit. Baked potato with the skin on is high in fiber.

Drink pure water, as much as six to eight glasses daily. When you take herbs and fiber supplements, it isn't hard to drink that much water.

Thermos cooking is an excellent way to supply nutrients and fiber that are lacking in the typical American diet. Cooking in a thermos is a slow gentle way to use grains without destroying the B-complex vitamins and enzymes.

A wide-mouthed thermos is ideal. It makes the food easier to remove. You rinse the thermos first with boiling water and spoon in the rinsed grain. Then fill to the top with boiling pure water. Close the lid tightly and leave to cook overnight. There will be plenty of water-space to take care of expansion. Use the extra liquid to drink, it is full of enzymes and vitamins and will be healing for the digestive tract. For grains use 1/2 cup to 1 and 1/2 cups of boiling water. This works well with for a pint and half thermos. Wash the grain, pour in boiling water and leave a few minutes to heat both the grain and the thermos. Drain again, and leave the grain in the thermos. Fill to the top with boiling water, close the thermos tightly and leave overnight.

Mixed Grains: Mix the following grains: buckwheat, kamut, whole oats, hard wheat, rye and whole barley. Use 1/2 cup of the mixed grain with 1 and 1/2 cup of boiling water.

Whole Wheat: Use 1/2 cup wheat to 1 and 1/2 cups water. For a quart thermos use 1 cup of wheat to 3 cups of water.

Brown Rice and Millet: This makes a nice breakfast. These need to be cooked in boiling water and simmered for five minutes before putting in the thermos. This helps to break the hard hulls so they are tender.

NUTRITIONAL SUPPLEMENTS

Acidophilus is used to increase good bacteria in the colon. It also helps in the digestion of food.

Food Digestive Enzymes are needed to break down toxins and foreign matter in the body. They aid in purifying the body.

Hydrochloric Acid Supplements (HCL) usually decline after the age of forty, but is seen in the young because of dietary habits. Is essential in the body to make the proper chemical conversion to alkalinity. Eight essential amino acids, vitamins and minerals need HCL for absorption. It destroys bacteria, germs and viruses. It also neutralizes parasites, worms and many toxins we ingest and breathe.

Blue-green Algae and Chlorophyll contain amino acids, which are healing for the cells and tissues. They increase oxygen utilization, provide nutrients and protect against viral disease.

Lower Bowel Formula restores bowel function by cleansing, nourishing and rebuilding the colon walls. The formula should contain cascara sagrada, barberry, buckthorn, raspberry leaves, ginger, lobelia, goldenseal, fennel, and cayenne.

Liver Herbal Formula is necessary to purify toxins from the blood. It should contain milk thistle, dandelion root, red beet root, goldenseal, yellow dock, bayberry, Oregon grape and lobelia.

Blood Herbal Formula is needed to neutralize acids and toxins from the blood. It should contain red clover, buckthorn bark, burdock, licorice, peach bark, prickly ash bark, echinacea, cascara, and sheep sorrel. The extract is absorbed directly into the bloodstream.

Vitamin and Mineral Supplements are essential to heal and restore proper function to the colon. B-complex vitamins help detoxify toxins, "bad" estrogen and balance hormones.

Vitamin C and bioflavonoids help to clean the veins.

Calcium and Magnesium are needed for strong nerves and heart.

Antioxidants protect against free-radical damage. These include vitamins A, C, E, the minerals selenium, zinc and grapeseed extract.

Cat's Claw contains anti-inflammatory properties. It is very healing for the digestive tract. It has the ability to clean up long-standing conditions of the digestive tract.

Facts at a glance

- Autointoxication is the cause of most diseases.
- Lack of fiber contributes to toxic colon.
- Diet devoid of enzymes causes toxins to thrive.
- Fasting on juices and herbal formulas increases detoxification of crusted colon.
- Lack of HCI causes an increase of bacteria, germs, viruses, worms and parasites. We may see more diseases with the new advertised antacids on the market.

Constipation/Toxic Buildup

Constipation is probably the least understood condition of the body and the most common problem with which people are plagued.

Over ninety percent of human ailments begin with a congested colon. Even if you eliminate three times a day you could still be constipated. Lack of dietary fiber is one of the main causes. The average American ingests white flour and white sugar products, a diet high in meat and fried food, with very little raw vegetables and fruit, and little or no whole grains. With this type of diet there will be problems in the bowel area. A congested colon will balloon and create pockets and weaken the walls of the colon, allowing bacterial toxins to enter the bloodstream and cause autointoxication.

Intestinal toxemia or autointoxication is produced by the decomposition of protein in the intestinal tract. In normal digestion the protein molecules are broken down into twenty amino acids. The amino acids are non-toxic; however under the influence of bacterial growth they are capable of producing amines, which are highly poisonous and found in a toxic colon.

A congested colon causes the poisons to be reabsorbed in the bloodstream and settle in the weakest areas of the body to eventually cause chronic diseases. These toxins back up into the veins, arteries and lymphatic system and into the cells.

Diarrhea

Diarrhea can be a form of constipation. Dr. John Christopher says that, "diarrhea is simply a bad condition in the intestinal tract, where it is so badly clogged that the fecal solids are being held back and only the eliminative liquids are getting through."

Diarrhea is caused by an irritation in the colon. Chronic diarrhea is caused when the irritating substance is glued to the walls of the colon and cannot be eliminated. A lower bowel herbal formula will gradually peel off the hardened crust on the colon walls.

All diarrhea isn't necessarily constipation. The following can cause diarrhea: food poisoning, parasites, flu, colds, anxiety and conditions such as Crohn's disease, ulcerative colitis, diverticular disease, irritable bowel syndrome or cancer of the large intestine.

Normal laxatives on the market are harmful and habit-forming. They work against nature, and pull liquids and minerals from the body, creating more damage in the long run.

Lower bowel herbal formulas are excellent in assisting nature to clean, nourish, rebuild and restore the bowel's normal function. Herbs work on the root of the problem. With a cleansing diet, and then adding raw vegetables and fruit, brown rice and whole grains, the bowels can be restored to normal function.

Most people have pounds of dried fecal matter that are stored in the colon, preventing food from being digested and assimilated. Because of this, many people eat more food than the body requires, trying to get sufficient nutrition and yet they are still hungry. It may take months to restore the lower bowel area, but by using herbs, food will assimilate better. A person can sustain herself on less food, with more energy and vitality than was thought possible.

Dr. Arbuthnot Lane

In 1929 Dr. Arbuthnot Lane, a well-respected English physician and colon specialist, made the dramatic statement that constipation was the cause of all the ills of civilization. Dr. Lane had worked for years as a surgeon who continually dealt with bowel problems. His "hands on" experience in repeatedly removing sections of diseased bowels provided him with impressive data and a firsthand look at the profound role of the colon in overall health.

One of the most striking correlations he discovered was between a malfunctioning colon and seemingly unrelated diseases. He noticed this particular phenomenon when some of his patients, who were recovering from colonic surgery, experienced remarkable cures in other parts of their bodies that had no apparent connection to the colon.

One young boy had suffered from such serious arthritis for several years that at the time of his colon surgery was confined to a wheelchair. Six months after the colon surgery, he experienced a complete recovery from the arthritis. Another female patient who had suffered with a goiter, showed signs of remission within six months of her colonic surgery. Dr Lane was intrigued and subsequently discovered a long list of diseases, ranging from tuberculosis to rheumatism which were cured when certain diseased sections of the bowel were removed. He found that specific areas of the colon affected certain body organs.

Dr. Lane was so impressed with the notion that a toxic bowel could determine the health of other body systems, he completely changed his methods of medical treatment. He spent the last twenty-five years of this life dedicated to teaching people how to care for the colon through proper nutrition, thereby avoiding the risk of bowel surgery. He emphasized the importance of transit time or how long waste material is retained in the colon and stated, "The lower end of the intestine is the size that requires emptying every six hours, but by habit, we retain its content twenty-four hours. The result is ulcers, cancer and other diseases."

SYMPTOMS

• enlarged abdomen, with discomfort
• headaches
• depression, anxiety, irritability
• fatigue and exhaustion
• indigestion and gas
• insomnia, and frequent waking up in the night
• overweight, malnutrition, glandular imbalance
• lower back pain (colon pressing on sciatic nerve)
• skin, hair and nail problems

CAUSES

Lack of fiber in the diet slows the elimination of fecal matter, allowing toxins to infect colon pockets. Adhesions can be a cause of constipation due to infected mucous membranes of the bowel wall. Other causes include: a stretched colon from overload of food contents; ileocecal valve incompetence, which allows bowel content to re-enter the small intestine and damage organs, joints, nerves and the immune system; and lack of exercise, especially in the abdominal area.

Poor posture interfering with the voluntary and reflex contractions of these important muscles necessary for normal elimination; constipation causes hemorrhoids, and hemorrhoids cause spasms or tightness of the anal muscle and prevents normal bowel elimination; weak bowel muscles can become paralyzed and prevent complete emptying of the bowels. This allows toxins from the fecal matter to irritate the mucous membranes and produce chronic catarrhal, infections, adhesions and even cancer. Lack of liquids causes dehydration, which creates hard fecal matter and prevents normal elimination. Lack of water is usually the cause. Lack of hydrochloric acid and digestive enzymes can eventually lead to constipation and autointoxication.

How We Become Constipated

The lack of fiber and eating large amounts of mucus-forming food causes the body to produce excess amounts of mucus to protect the intestines from absorbing toxins. This mucus medium develops and slows the transit time through the colon walls. This causes the contents to remain in the colon longer than it should. Moisture is pulled from the contents and becomes packed together and hardens on the intestinal walls. If a lot of fat and white flour products are eaten it causes a glue-like substance to stick to the colon walls. As this glue-like material hardens it builds up on the colon walls layer after layer and becomes rubbery and hard. The pockets of the colon collect this hard material and causes such strong adherence it does not pass from the body with the daily bowel eliminations.

Too much mucus is also produced when large amounts of cooked foods are eaten, especially food such as meat, cheese, milk products, pastries, candy, white flour products, white pasta and all processed food. These are called glue-foods.

We have learned that when cooked food is eaten the T-cells come to the rescue because it sees food without enzymes as a foreign invader. This puts a burden on the immune system, eventually weakening it. Mucus is also formed to protect the body from poisons. If cooked and processed food is eaten day after day without raw food and fiber, the contents eventually build up on the colon walls like rings around a tree.

This causes the immune system to become overworked and creates a medium for germs, viruses, parasites and worms to invade the body. Autoimmune diseases develop because the immune system is confused and overworked and begins to attack the body. We have overstimulated and overworked the immune and digestive systems and they can no longer protect us.

NATURAL TREATMENT

Lifestyle changes need to be made. Eliminate alcohol, tobacco, carbonated drinks, white flour and white sugar products and greasy food. Increase dietary fiber, raw foods and reduce meat and fat. This will decrease the accumulation of bad bacteria while building and protecting the immune system.

Exercise is also very important, especially for the abdominal area. Jumping on a mini-trampoline and walking are good exercises. Using a rowing machine and squatting exercises will strengthen the abdomen and intestinal system.

Learn to listen to the inner body and eat only when hungry. Avoid eating when you are emotionally upset. Learn to combine foods that digest well together. Combining meat and sugar and starch will cause fermentation and create an alcohol substance in the stomach and intestines. Learn about your own body and your particular weaknesses and what nutrients will build and maintain physical, emotional and mental health.

Eliminate over-the-counter laxatives, as they interfere with the proper absorption of sodium and potassium balance in the large intestine. Laxatives pull water and minerals from the body.

DIETARY GUIDELINES

Add more whole grains such as whole wheat, whole oats, brown rice, millet, kamut, buckwheat, yellow corn meal (polenta dishes are delicious), amaranth, quinoa, and spelt. Whole grains provide fiber, the fatty acids, B-vitamins and minerals when in their whole state. Cooking in a slow cooker or thermos overnight is very nutritional. Chew food longer to assure enzyme activity and help to prevent constipation. Chewing longer satisfies hunger and prevents indigestion.

Juice fasting for one to three days will help start a cleansing of the bowels. Good juice combinations are: carrot, celery, parsley and garlic; and cabbage, carrots, celery and ginger. Wheatgrass juice is cleansing for the colon and blood. Some have benefited from a wheatgrass and garlic enema to speed colon cleansing.

A liver flush is very beneficial with all the toxins in our water, food and air. First thing in the morning, mix in blender one cup warm water, juice of one lime or lemon, 1 capsule ginger or 1 teaspoon fresh ginger, and one teaspoon pure olive oil. Mix and drink. This will clean and stimulate liver function.

A fresh juice made with grapefruit, oranges, limes and lemons drink before breakfast will aid the body in cleansing.

A fiber and herbal formula is beneficial for cleansing deep into the pockets of the colon. It should contain psyllium, guar gum, burdock, black walnut and pumpkin seeds.

Make flaxseed tea by soaking a tablespoon of flaxseeds in a quart of pure water overnight. Mix in the blender, strain, and drink a cup twice a day.

Plain yogurt, made from live culture, is very nourishing for the bowels. It provides friendly bacteria in the bowels and builds immunity to disease.

Nutritional Supplements

Lower Bowel Herbal Formula should contain some of the following: cascara sagrada, red raspberry, barberry, lobelia, ginger, goldenseal, fennel and cayenne. This formula is designed to clean, nourish, and restore natural bowel function. These are herbal foods for the small and large bowels. This is not considered a true laxative, but is developed to clean and rebuild.

Hydrochloric Acid is necessary to break down protein into amino acids for proper digestion. It destroys bacteria, germs, viruses, parasites and worms. It is essential for life, and the only acid our body produces. It breaks down food to prevent undigested waste residue from entering the bloodstream, and causing toxins to damage the cells.

Plant Digestive Enzymes are essential to help break down any undigested food in the transverse colon where putrefaction occurs when food remains too long in that area. They improve elimination and neutralize the odor in stools.

Digestive Enzymes should contain protease, which breaks down protein. Lipase breaks down fat; amylase breaks down starch; cellulase assists to break down cellulose. Digestive enzymes will also clean out the blood and cells of protein lodged anywhere in the body.

Acidophilus is used to protect the body from bad bacteria. Necessary to use when cleansing the colon. Also will help in the digestion of food.

Blue-green Algae and Chlorophyll increase oxygen utilization, provide nutrients and protect against viral diseases.

Liver Herbal Formula helps to detoxify and nourish the liver. It should contain milk thistle, dandelion, red beet root, goldenseal, yellow dock, bayberry, Oregon grape and lobelia.

Amino Acid combination helps restore proper function to the bowels. Histidine and glycine promote natural secretions of stomach acid, and also increase saliva production in the mouth. Amino acids are healing and will digest and assimilate properly.

Vitamin A is needed to heal and nourish the tissues.

Antioxidants, like vitamins A, C, E, and minerals selenium and zinc supply oxygen and carry nutrients needed to support mucous membrane linings. They also help prevent leaky gut syndrome.

B-complex vitamins help regulate and eliminate toxins in the liver. They are especially essential for balancing and eliminating "bad" estrogen from the liver. They are also needed for nervous system disorders and depression.

Indoles increase the activity of enzymes, destroy toxins and may also change the hormone estrogen into a benign form. They have the ability to block cancer-causing substances before they enter the cells. They are also found in cruciferous vegetables. (However, supplements are stronger).

Herbs that are nourishing to the colon are: aloe vera, which is a natural laxative and helps to dissolve adhesions; ginger, which prevents cramping and stimulates bile secretions to help in excretion of small gallstones and relieve constipation; black walnut, which eliminates worms; burdock, which neutralizes toxins and cleans the blood; goldenseal, which kills parasites and heals the colon; and slippery elm, which heals the colon.

Essential Fatty Acids (flaxseed oil, evening primrose, borage, black currant, salmon oil) are essential for every function of the body. They work with vitamin E to help prevent heart attacks and strokes.

Cat's Claw is an excellent herb found to have the ability to clear and cleanse the entire intestinal tract. It contains anti-inflammatory properties, which are vital for treating diseases such as arthritis and allergies. Some believe it has anti-viral and immune activity more effective than both echinacea and pau d'arco.

FACTS AT A GLANCE

• Constipation can cause chronic diseases.
• Lack of fiber is one of the main causes of constipation.
• Enzymes and amino acids are very helpful in cleaning the cells and blood, and to break down protein to be eliminated.
• An herbal lower bowel cleanser will gradually clean and restore colon health.
• A change of diet will help restore colon function.

Crohn's Disease

Approximately two million Americans suffer from Crohn's disease and ulcerative colitis. These are diseases which come under the title of inflammatory bowel disease (IBD). This disease is becoming more and more common — this is significant because if it is left untreated, it can lead to cancer. Crohn's disease is an inflammation of any portion of the gastrointestinal tract and extends through all layers of the intestinal wall.

SYMPTOMS

• diarrhea
• abdominal pain
• rectal bleeding
• anemia
• weight loss
• abdominal infections
• low stress tolerance

Causes

Doctors are puzzled as to the cause of this sickness. However, there is speculation by some of the medical profession that it is related to allergies, other immune disorders, or an overburdened lymphatic system. The medical profession treats it with steroids and antibiotics. When medical therapy is not effective, surgical removal of the diseased area may be necessary.

It is felt that Crohn's disease is an "autoimmune" disorder. The digestive tract is overtaxed with the constant eating of cooked food without enzymes to break it down. The body becomes so toxic from many years of toxin buildup from medications and poor eating habits that the immune system becomes confused. It then attacks the toxic tissues, and begins to destroy them, thinking they are a foreign organism. Another cause or result of Crohn's disease is parasite infestation, which further debilitates the immune system.

Natural Treatment

It takes a diligent program of certain herbs and diet to get rid of parasites and heal the digestive tract. But first we must eliminate the garbage on which they feed: mucus-producing "foods" such as refined pastries, partially digested meat, dairy products and all junk food. These products contribute to the "slime" on which the microbes thrive. A person with Crohn's disease has severe digestive problems and the foods above are difficult to digest. Also when a person is under stress (this disease causes stress on the body), and eats cooked food they do not digest properly. This causes weakness and a person can become malnourished because the few nutrients they do get are not assimilated.

People with Crohn's disease need to cleanse, eliminate parasites, work with digestion and build the immune system. These steps will enable the body to begin the job of repairing the damage. The body will heal itself, given the proper tools.

Dietary Guidelines

Adding digestive enzymes is the first step to healing. First of all they will help break down the undigested protein, toxins, and parasites so they can be eliminated and take the burden off the immune system.

Juice fasting will take the burden off the digestive system, supply nutrients and heal the GI tract. Carrot, cabbage, parsley, and ginger taken together will heal. A juice combination of carrot, celery, endive and garlic is healing.

An herbal fiber formula will heal and clean the pockets of the colon. It should contain psyllium and guar gum. Dietary fiber is usually well-tolerated. Fruit, vegetables, grains, and almond and sesame milk will help heal the digestive tract.

Vegetable soups are healing, as they are rich in minerals. No healing can take place without minerals. An herbal mineral drink, high in potassium, will heal the mucous membranes. Potassium is essential for good digestion. Use garlic and ginger in the soups; they will heal and kill parasites. Millet is easy to digest, and is healing and high in minerals, especially calcium and magnesium.

Cook grains and vegetables in a thermos. Add pure water and drink the juice, it is rich in enzymes for healing. Well-tolerated foods are brown rice, millet, sweet potatoes, winter squash, non-citrus fruits and yellow and green vegetables.

Nutritional Supplements

Aloe Vera Juice heals inflammation, enhances digestion, cleans the colon, and heals adhesions.

Acidophilus heals, helps the body digest food, and protects from bad bacteria.

Blue-green Algae and Chlorophyll are rich in minerals, and are cleansing and healing for the digestive tract. Wheatgrass is also healing.

Slippery Elm is healing and nourishing for the digestive tract. It is soothing while restoring normal function.

Goldenseal and Capsicum are excellent for healing internal bleeding and inflammation.

Licorice Root has antiviral properties and is healing for the digestive tract.

Herbs to eliminate parasites include goldenseal, black walnut, senna, and wormwood. Yellow dock kills the parasite larva, which is important, in order to prevent chances of reinfestation. Bugleweed also kills larva.

Germanium and Co Q-10 fortify the immune system and aid in healing damaged tissues, due to their oxygenation properties.

Cat's Claw cleans the intestinal tract. Contains anti-inflammatory and healing properties.

Red Clover Herbal Formula will clean and heal the blood and digestive tract. It should contain red clover, buckthorn, burdock, echinacea, licorice, prickly ash and sheep sorrel.

Nervine Formula should contain skullcap, passion flower, wild yam, hops or valerian root, and St. John's wort.

Facts At A Glance

• Crohn's disease is seen in countries where high amounts of meat, dairy products and white sugar and flour products are consumed.

• Increasing fiber is beneficial in cleaning the intestines.

• Nutritional supplements and change of diet will alter the environment of the bowel area.

• Positive attitude and using nervine herbs will help in the healing of the entire body.

Diverticulitis

Diverticulitis is a common and serious disease of the intestines. Fiber (the indigestible part of food) helps the muscle contractions of the walls of the intestines. It increases peristaltic action to draw food quickly through the alimentary canal.

When food moves too slowly through the alimentary canal, the hard elimination and undigested food causes pouches to form on the intestinal wall. These are called diverticula. These pouches become filled with toxic feces which cause irritation and infections. This is caused by poor bowel function and autointoxication. Also, undigested protein can leak through the intestinal wall and cause all kinds of diseases. Autoimmune diseases are increased with bowel problems such as leaky gut syndrome.

SYMPTOMS

- cramping in the abdomen
- tenderness on the left side
- fever from infection
- constipation alternating with diarrhea
- nausea and vomiting
- abdominal swelling
- cramps and pain
- hemorrhaging and rectal bleeding

CAUSES

Constipation and straining from hard stools cause the diverticuli to develop. It can be serious and develop into cancer if left untreated. Stress is put on the nerves and body when constipation throws toxins back into the bloodstream and causes irritations to the brain and nerves. Poor eating habits are a big factor in causing this disease. Lack of fiber is the main cause.

This disease causes malnutrition because of poor digestion and absorption. It causes improper secretion of saliva in the mouth and prevents proper digestion and enzyme processes. Cataracts are formed, and hearing is impaired because the organs are starved of nutrition and oxygen.

NATURAL TREATMENT

A high-fiber diet using whole grains, vegetables, fruit, beans, sprouts, and almonds will provide natural bulk to clean the colon. This disease has developed rapidly in the last fifty years, and emerged when whole grains were replaced by white flour products, increased meat and dairy products and the wide use of white sugar products in the diet.

Soothing herbs will help heal the intestinal tract. Slippery elm is healing and soothing. Garlic enemas will help infections.

DIETARY GUIDELINES

Juice fasting is one of the quickest ways to heal the digestive system. Use carrots, celery, endive and garlic. Juice, and drink immediately for best results. Another nutritious combination is carrots, celery, parsley and cabbage or green pepper.

Digestive enzymes will help break down the undigested protein, toxins and parasites so they can be eliminated and will take the burden off the immune system.

Dietary fiber is usually well-tolerated. Fruit, vegetables, grains, and almond and sesame milk will help heal the digestive tract. An herbal fiber formula will heal and clean the pockets of the colon. It should contain psyllium and guar gum.

Plain yogurt containing live culture will speed the healing of the intestines. Add acidophilus to the yogurt.

Vegetable soups are healing; they are rich in minerals. Cook the following vegetables and use the broth to begin with: cabbage, potatoes with the skins, carrots, celery, onions, parsley, garlic and ginger. An herbal mineral drink, high in potassium, will heal the mucous membranes. Potassium is essential for good digestion.

Add millet and brown rice to the diet. Well-tolerated foods are sweet potatoes, winter squash, non-citrus fruits and green vegetables.

NUTRITIONAL SUPPLEMENTS

Herbal fiber formulas will heal and help clean the pockets of the colon wall. It should contain psyllium husk and guar gum to clean out the pockets. Papaya, fenugreek, slippery elm, ginger and marshmallow, will heal, soothe and clean the colon. The combination of black walnut and pumpkin seed powder will eliminate parasites and worms. Echinacea and garlic will heal infections. Aloe vera is healing, and capsicum will stop any bleeding.

Acidophilus is necessary for restoring the friendly bacteria; it also helps in the digestion of food.

Aloe Vera Juice is healing and helps in preventing scarring.

Vitamin A heals the mucous membranes and protects against infections.

Vitamin E is healing and prevents scarring.

B-complex Vitamins are necessary for a healthy digestive tract. They also strengthens the nervous system.

Antioxidants are healing; Vitamins A, E, C, and minerals selenium and zinc, and grapeseed extract are among the best.

Minerals are necessary for healing and protecting the lining of the colon.

Essential Fatty Acids protect the cells and nourish the glands and the entire body.

Amino Acid Supplement will help speed the healing of the digestive tract.

Plant Digestive Enzymes help in the breakdown of undigested protein in the cells and blood. They will also help speed healing.

Cat's Claw has strong healing properties and helps in inflammation.

FACTS AT A GLANCE

• Diverticulitis develops from lack of fiber in the diet.

• Constipation causes pockets to develop because of straining from hard stools.

• Nutrients and fasting will help heal the digestive tract.

• Digestive enzymes will help in eliminating the cause of irritation to the digestive tract.

Irritable Bowel Syndrome

Stress seems to be the main cause of IBS, but now there is evidence that it is more than stress. Actually, bad diet, undigested food and a toxic colon contribute to IBS, and all this puts stress on the body. A toxic colon can put stress on the nerves and brain.

IBS is an inflammatory disease of the intestinal tract and affects the large intestine. Women suffer from IBS more than men. It is a result of poorly digested food, creating toxins and mucus in the bloodstream which irritates the lower bowels.

Symptoms

• abdominal pain
• alternating constipation and diarrhea (both from an irritated and congested colon)
• bloating and gas (which could be from yeast infection)
• depression
• nausea
• fatigue (from diarrhea, which can cause loss of minerals)

Causes

A low-fiber diet is the main cause of IBS. This allows toxins to irritate the intestines. A congested liver is associated with IBS. Cooked fats and oils contribute to liver congestion, and slows digestion and transit time of food. Toxins in the colon promote the retention of "bad" estrogens that fuel the growth of tumors in the uterus, breast and ovaries and all female reproductive areas.

A diet high in meat, dairy products, white flour and sugar products and fried food, all contribute to IBS.

Natural Treatment

A change in eating habits is the first line of defense. This will start the healing process of the intestines. A diet high in fiber such as whole grains, vegetables and fruit will help heal and restore intestinal health.

Relaxation therapy, exercise, and a positive attitude help contribute to the overall health of the body. Learning to accept changes, and let go of the past will help in colon health. The Chinese feel that the large intestine is associated with grief, and if we let go of the past, colon health will improve. Many women have improved their emotions by improving their colon health.

Exercises such as squatting, jumping on a trampoline or using a rowing machine improve the lower bowel function.

DIETARY GUIDELINES

Juice fasting will help heal the intestines. Juices supply vitamins, minerals and enzymes necessary for colon health. Examples include the combination of carrot, celery, parsley, and ginger. Cabbage, endive, carrot and celery are healing.

A natural electrolyte replacement drink will prevent loss of nutrients that usually accompany diarrhea. Add a protein drink that contains all the essential amino acids or use an amino acid supplement.

NUTRITIONAL SUPPLEMENTS

Acidophilus increases friendly bacteria in the colon and also aids digestion.

Plant Digestive Enzymes help to eliminate the parasites, protein and toxins that can irritate the colon. Properly digested food will prevent undigested residue in the blood and cells.

Blue-green Algae is healing and nourishing for the colon.

High-Fiber Supplements increase bulk, which help cleanse the pockets of the colon and eliminate trapped food.

Lower Bowel Formula heals, nourishes and cleans the large intestine.

Herbal Nervine Formula is necessary to build up and restore health to the nerves and brain. It should contain passion flower, hops, skullcap, valerian root, amino acids.

Vitamin and mineral supplements are needed to nourish the body and strengthen the immune system.

Cat's Claw has the power to heal the intestines.

FACTS AT A GLANCE

- Irritable bowel syndrome is caused from a toxic colon.
- Lack of enzymes causes a buildup of undigested protein in the tissues. Food lodges in the pockets of the colon and causes irritations.
- A high-fiber diet will help heal and restore bowel function.
- A change of diet and exercise can help in IBS.

Section 3

The Urinary System

If there is but little water in the stream, it is the fault, not of the channel, but of the source.

ST. JEROME

The Body's Waterworks

The kidneys are constantly working. A consistent drip occurs day in and day out, all day and all night (three to four times more by day than by night) from the kidneys into the bladder. The kidneys are the chief organs for cleansing the body's internal fluid. They comprise our filtering system, and they absorb and excrete toxins. If the filters are plugged up, it may cause infections, and when the kidneys lose their ability to filter toxins and the blood, they can become diseased and cause loss of protein in the blood, which is, in turn, lost in the urine. Weak kidneys will also lose essential nutrients such as potassium, calcium, magnesium and zinc. Kidney disease causes toxins to remain in the blood and poison the tissues. Kidney failure can cause high blood pressure, stroke, heart attack or glaucoma.

The kidneys' job is to maintain a constant and healthy internal environment in the body. They adjust the body's electrolyte balance. They manufacture hormones that regulate blood pressure, calcium metabolism and red blood cell production. The kidneys are very efficient. They eliminate whatever is bad for the body and brain and any excess of the good. If you go on a candy spree, sugar rises in the blood, reaches a concentration too high for safety, and the kidneys have the job of throwing out the excess.

The kidneys try to maintain the health of the body, but when pain, pallor, swelling, high blood pressure, blood in the urine, burning and stinging occur, you know your kidneys are in trouble.

Toxins can accumulate in the blood and cause kidney damage. Alcohol, drugs and smoking, as well as exposure to heavy metals such as cadmium, lead and mercury, can cause damage to the kidneys. These can accumulate and cause harm. Drinking water and air pollution contain metals. Smokers have higher incidences of kidney failure than nonsmokers.

About 12 million Americans experience urinary incontinence, and it affects all ages, not just the elderly. There are many diseases, as well as pregnancy, infections, surgery, and obesity, that can cause this condition.

Kidney stones are common and about 90 percent are caused by calcium deposits. The concentration of calcium can be eliminated without surgery. Distilled water, herbal calcium products, and formulas to heal and strengthen the kidneys are helpful.

Bladder and Kidney Infections

The urinary system plays a critical role in the inner health and cleanliness of the body. The kidneys are the purification filters for the blood. The body depends on the kidneys to remove potentially toxic chemicals that are in the bloodstream. They also regulate the fluid and electrolyte balance in the body.

Symptoms

• cloudy, dark-colored or scanty urine
• continuous, dull pain in the lower abdomen or lower back
• burning sensation during urination
• feeling the need for frequent urination
• chills and fever

Causes

Infections and inflammations are fairly common, especially in the bladder and urethra. (Cystitis is the name for infections in this area.) They are usually caused by bacteria but can be caused by chemical irritants in soaps, bubble bath, talcum powder, perfumes or vaginal deodorants. These can cause inflammation in the urethra. Sexual intercourse can also cause cystitis, by bruising the urethra, introducing infection-causing bacteria and setting up an inflammation process. (For this reason it is sometimes referred to as "honeymoon cystitis.") Yeast overgrowth can also cause cystitis. Infections can cause incontinence (the inability to control urination).

Frequent urination can be a symptom of a disease such as diabetes. Difficult urination can be caused by a urethral stricture. Kidney problems can cause pain in the lower back. The bladder holds the urine and if toxins accumulate without being eliminated often, it can develop infections. Drinking plenty of pure water will help keep the bladder clean.

Autointoxication is one cause of bladder and kidney infections. Constipation causes a back-up of toxins in the bloodstream, which irritates the bladder. Congested kidneys will cause the skin to try and eliminate these poisons. The skin is the largest elimination organ of the body and takes over if the kidneys are plugged up with mucus material and toxins. The liver helps to detoxify and clean the blood and convert toxins into water-soluble particles. The kidneys are the filters that collect toxic particles and pass them out of the body. Donald LePore, N.D., states in his book, *The Ultimate Healing System,*

Many doctors believe that a high calcium intake will cause kidney problems. This in part is true, because if there is not enough magnesium to work with the calcium, there will be problems. So, instead of limiting a person's calcium intake (except at the very beginning of the problem), the best thing for you to do is to administer magnesium, which is the controller of calcium, in order to dissolve kidney stones and calcification.

Most kidney infections are not infections, but inflammations, unless there has been an accident or blow to the kidneys. Kidney stones and calcification are usually non-functional causes of kidney disease. Pains in the back below the lower ribs are usually a tell-tale sign that calcification or other problems are starting

KIDNEY STONES

A fast using pure apple juice alternating with lemon or lime juice will soften kidney stones. This can be done for three days. Before retiring drink 1/4 cup of pure olive oil in a cup of warm water with a capsule of licorice, ginger and fenugreek. Open the capsules and blend all together and drink. Aloe vera juice will also help soften kidney stones.

NATURAL TREATMENT

Juice fasting will help the kidneys and bladder. Liquid chlorophyll will purify the blood. Pure apple juice, green drinks and citrus juices will cleanse and heal. Enemas or lower bowel cleansers in herbal formulas will also help eliminate toxins from the system. Wear underwear that allows air circulation (cotton is best). Toilet tissue should be used from the front to the back to prevent irritations and infections.

DIETARY GUIDELINES

Eat a high-fiber diet. Constipation can cause irritations from a toxic build-up in the blood. Consume milk products sparingly; they will produce an acid condition. Foods like garlic, onions, potassium broths (potato peelings, carrot tops, parsley, celery, etc.), cherry juice or fresh lemon juice in pure water (one-half lemon at a time) is healing. It acts as a natural antiseptic and helps to destroy bacteria. Unsweetened cranberry juice or powdered cranberry in capsules is very powerful. Cranberry contains properties that prevent bacteria from adhering to the walls of the bladder. Michael Murray discussed the benefits of cranberry, saying

> Cranberries and cranberry juice have been used to treat bladder infections and have proved to be quite effective in several clinical studies. In one study of patients with active urinary tract infections, drinking 16 ounces of cranberry juice per day was shown to produce beneficial effects in 73 percent of the subjects (44 females and 16 males). . . . Furthermore, withdrawal of the supplemental cranberry juice from the diets of those who had benefited resulted in recurrence of bladder infection in 61 percent." (Michael Murray, *The Healing Power of Foods*. Rocklin, CA: Prima Publishing, 1993, p. 139)

A fast to clean the blood would be beneficial, using fresh juices if possible or frozen, followed by a low-mucus-forming diet (low-meat, low-fat; primarily fresh fruits and vegetables). High-protein diets causes calcium to accumulate in the kidneys (and thus depriving other areas of calcium), leading to kidney stones. Excess protein is broken down by the liver and kidneys, so it would be best to not overwork these organs. A good protein source would be free-form amino acids for easier assimilation. Vegetable proteins are the best. Drink at least one gallon of reverse osmosis purified water daily. Watermelon is very beneficial for cleansing the kidneys and bladder. Marshmallow and slippery elm also help if there is bleeding in the urinary tract. Parsley is a natural diuretic, and vitamins and is valuable for nephritis. Use soups with asparagus, celery, spinach and parsley with herb seasoning.

Things to avoid include carbonated beverages, black tea, coffee, alcohol and caffeine drinks and sugar products. These items may cause inflammation of the membranes lining the kidneys.

Nutritional Supplements

Buchu is highly esteemed for helping problems such as kidney inflammation caused by an acidic condition in the urine. It seems to assist increased urine flow, and cleans the kidneys of mucus buildup and toxins. Buchu is often recommended for treating urinary disorders such as bladder infections, inflammation, and painful urination. It is known to absorb the excess uric acid and toxins in the urine, relieving bladder irritations. It is also used for conditions such as cystitis, urethritis, and prostatitis. Buchu acts as a tonic, astringent and disinfectant on the mucous membranes. It is cleansing, strengthening and relaxing to the urinary system.

Garlic is one of nature's antibiotics. It has a rejuvenating effect on all body functions. Garlic stimulates the lymphatic system to cleanse the body of toxins. Even though it is effective against bacteria which may be resistant to antibiotic drugs, it does not destroy the body's normal flora.

Echinacea stimulates the immune system and increases the body's ability to resist infections. It helps remove toxins from the blood.

Goldenseal contains hydrastine, which acts like an antibiotic. It is a very healing and soothing herb for all mucous membranes in the body. It has a beneficial effect and contains tonic properties to help in all kidney problems. Goldenseal will help the body to build up natural immunity to kidney infections. It should not be used during pregnancy.

Hydrangea is considered useful for preventing kidney stones from forming. It helps relieve pain when the formations pass through the ureters from the kidney to the bladder.

Juniper Berries are excellent for clearing the blood of uric acid that is retained in the system. This plant helps eliminate yeast infections, as well as kidney infections. Juniper has a beneficial effect on the kidneys and helps to counteract urine retention, stones, pain, bladder discharges and uric acid buildup.

Parsley has a positive effect on the kidneys, bladder, stomach, liver and gallbladder. It is a great preventative herb, and is especially useful combined with marshmallow. It has a tonic effect on the entire urinary tract and should be used as a preventive aid in kidney infections. It is a very effective diuretic. It should not be used in medicinal dosages during pregnancy, as there may be excessive stimulation of the uterus.

Cranberries help prevent bacteria from adhering to the walls of the bladder.

Uva Ursi strengthens and tones the urinary passages. It is especially beneficial for bladder and kidney infections. It increases the flow of urine and is useful for inflammatory diseases of the urinary tract, including cystitis. It should not be used during pregnancy in any large quantities because of the possibility of decreased circulation to the fetus.

Vitamins A and C protect against bladder infections and disease. Vitamin C with bioflavonoids helps prevent the accumulation of toxins in the bladder.

A deficiency of choline (found in lecithin) has been found to lead to kidney damage.

A deficiency of potassium can lead to renal disorders and kidney infections.

Chlorophyll cleans and nourishes the kidneys and bladder.

Magnesium and vitamin B6 help prevent kidney stones.

Acidophilus helps prevent infections.

FACTS AT A GLANCE

- Drink plenty of pure water to flush kidneys and bladder of toxins.
- High-protein diets are hard on the kidneys.
- Eat plenty of fresh fruits and vegetables.
- Take key supplements to ensure the health of the urinary system.

Section 4

The Respiratory System

As steam moves the wheels of the locomotive, so Air moves the Wheels of Life.

ANONYMOUS

The Vital Breath of Life

The brain is dependent upon every breath we take for its survival, and the breath of life begins with healthy lungs. Every cell and tissue of the body require oxygen to function properly. Breathing is such an automatic function that we do not think about it until we have a problem such as asthma or emphysema.

The respiratory system is comprised of the nose, mouth, pharynx, trachea, bronchii and lungs. (The pharynx is the throat; the trachea is the tube in the neck which begins at the larynx, or voice box, and ends at the top of the lungs, where the trachea then divides into two bronchii which extend into the lungs.) The respiratory system makes sure the body inhales oxygen and exhales carbon dioxide as a waste product. When we inhale, the air is warmed by the throat and travels down to the trachea and then the lungs. It is processed by air sacs called alveoli and pulmonary capillaries. Oxygen and carbon dioxide are then taken by the blood and distributed to the cells and tissues of the body. However, most of the carbon dioxide is removed from the body by the lungs and kidneys. We need to keep our respiratory system in healthy shape because our existence depends upon it.

Respiratory Diseases

Respiratory diseases can occur as asthma, bronchitis, emphysema, pneumonia, pleurisy or tuberculosis. The lungs are one of the channels of elimination. The lungs and the kidneys expel the greatest percentage of worn-out phosphorus and all waste material is removed from the cells through proper breathing.

The lungs are also weakened when the typical American diet is eaten. It causes colon congestion and autointoxication, and when the kidneys and colon become overloaded the lungs take over. The lungs are not meant to eliminate for other organs but it is the body's way of trying to protect us. The delicate lungs become irritated, weak and susceptible to germs, viruses, and bacteria.

Cigarette smoking causes lung diseases such as cancer, bronchitis, emphysema, and tuberculosis. The inhaled smoke irritates the airways and lining of the lungs. The delicate air sacs in the lungs become covered with a sticky, black, tar. The lungs were not meant to breathe in toxic smoke. The irritation causes the tissues to produce excess mucus in order to protect the lungs. The toxins and mucus provide an atmosphere for bacteria, germs and viruses to multiply, increasing the risk for lung diseases.

Smoking also causes coronary artery disease by increasing blood platelets and clot formations and can lead to stroke and heart attack. Nicotine increases the heartbeat and requires increased oxygen, but the carbon monoxide in the smoke limits the oxygen the blood can provide.

To keep our lungs healthy is a challenge with all the toxins in our air and indoor pollutants. The toxins in the air that hinder lung function include lead, carbon monoxide, nitrogen oxide, cadmium, sulfur oxides, and fine particulates (PM 10). Indoor pollutants are molds, bacteria, perfumes, pesticides, mothballs, formaldehyde, lead, paint, cleansers, and air fresheners.

Asbestos is a chemical that causes severe lung damage, such as asbestosis, bronchial cancer, and mesothelioma (cancer of the lining of the lungs and abdomen).

Symptoms

- frequent coughing or wheezing
- dyspnea (shortness of breath)
- frequent lung infections
- chest pain
- runny nose
- allergies

Causes

The accumulation of mucus from incomplete digestion (lack of digestive enzymes), a diet high in mucus-forming food and constipation can cause respiratory diseases. Mucus accumulates when food is not properly digested. Air and household pollution can further irritate lungs that are already congested with mucus. Another cause is not treating colds, flu and acute diseases naturally. Nature has provided a natural way to eliminate mucus by giving us colds, but when we suppress them with drugs, the membrane lining of the lungs and bronchial tubes plug up with thick mucus. Over the years the mucus hardens and solidifies. This sets the stage for chronic diseases.

Natural Treatment

One study on asthma patients — published in the *Journal of Asthma* in 1985 — investigated a vegetarian diet as a therapy for asthma. Twenty-four patients were involved, who had asthma for an average of 12 years. After four months on a vegetarian diet, 71 percent had improved and after a year, 92 percent had improved and were able to reduce or eliminate their medications.

Juice fasting will help the body eliminate mucus. Fresh citrus juices have the ability to dissolve hard mucus; among these are carrot, celery, endive and ginger, and wheatgrass. Use only purified or distilled water.

Exercise is important to strengthen lung capacity, along with a cleansing program, change of diet and the addition of herbs, vitamins, minerals and supplements to clean and heal the lungs.

DIETARY GUIDELINES

To clean the colon and lungs, fiber foods need to be added. An herbal fiber supplement will be beneficial, and should contain psyllium and guar gum. Brown rice, millet and whole oats are excellent. Apples, carrots, and cherries contain pectin, which benefits the colon.

Potato soups (using the skin), that contain vegetables such as onions, leeks, garlic, carrots, celery, broccoli, cabbage, and almost any vegetable will help in digestion. Start with the broth of the soup first, to start the healing process. Later, when the colon and lungs are stronger, eat the whole soup.

Just changing your diet will start the body to cleanse. If you change gradually it may not be too hard. Eliminate white flour products and foods cooked in oils; they act like glue on the colon and prevent proper digestion and assimilation. They also cause toxins to be absorbed into the blood and irritate the delicate lining of the lungs.

NUTRITIONAL SUPPLEMENTS

Vitamin A and E work together to heal and prevent lung diseases.

Vitamin C with bioflavonoids is needed every day to protect the lungs. It acts as a natural antihistamine and increases lung capacity. Low levels of vitamin C are seen in asthmatics.

B-complex Vitamins are necessary for digestion, and help liver to eliminate toxins. They are essential for a healthy nervous system.

Minerals are essential for lung health, and are needed for every function of the body. Those most valuable include calcium, iron, silicon, potassium, manganese and copper. Mineral supplements combined with herbs like alfalfa, dandelion, kelp and dulse are very good.

Plant Digestive Enzymes are necessary for breaking up and digesting toxins in the blood and cells. Use after eating and use between meals.

Hydrochloric Acid is necessary for the stomach to break down food. It protects the body against parasites, worms, viruses and toxins.

Germanium and Co Q-10 provide oxygen to the blood and cells.

Blue-green Algae and Chlorophyll are good for building and cleaning the blood, the colon and lungs.

Herbs to break up and eliminate mucus include boneset, elecampane, garlic, echinacea, lobelia, marshmallow, mullein, and myrrh.

Herbs with decongestant and expectorant properties include horehound, licorice, edphedra, pleurisy root, hyssop, eucalyptus, thyme, garlic, and blue vervain.

Herbs to neutralize toxins include blue-green algae, kelp, dulse, bee pollen, alfalfa, goldenseal, garlic, aloe vera, fenugreek, and lobelia.

Herbs to relax the nerves and body include skullcap, chamomile, passion flower, St. John's wort, licorice root, white willow, hops, valerian root, lady's slipper and wood betony.

Herbs with anti-inflammatory properties include alfalfa, marshmallow, butcher's broom and yarrow.

Herbs rich in nutrients for the lungs include alfalfa, kelp, dulse, plantain, blue-green algae, wheatgrass, kamut grass, barley grass, rose hips, and dandelion.

Facts at a Glance

- Congested colon releases gases, vapors and toxins in the bloodstream, which irritates the lungs.
- A vegetarian diet has helped people with lung diseases.
- Regular exercise will strengthen the lungs.
- Herbal formulas will clean, strengthen and nourish the lungs.

Colds, Flu, Fever, and Coughs

Colds, flu, fevers and all acute diseases are the body's natural attempt to clear the toxins from the body. When the body becomes so congested from bad eating habits, exhaustion and malnutrition it will cause an acute disease to develop, mainly to save one's life.

Frequent colds and flu are often caused from an imbalance in the colon, kidneys, liver, lymph, stomach and mucous membranes. Everyone is constantly in contact with germs, bacteria, viruses and air pollution, yet only those with an imbalance in the body come down with a cold or flu.

Dr. Henry Lindlahr, M.D., taught natural medicine at the turn of the century. He taught that all acute and chronic diseases must go through five stages of inflammation. This is based on "nature' law." Scientists all around the world spend millions of dollars seeking a cure for the common cold. They are trying to discover a drug to prevent and destroy the germs that cause and spread the common cold. They will never find a cure for the common cold. The cold, flu and all acute diseases are the cure. They are nature's efforts to eliminate from the body waste material, poisons, and to repair damage to healthy tissues. Every acute disease is the result of a cleansing and healing effort of nature. Some acute diseases are childhood diseases, asthma, bladder infections, croup, diarrhea, dysentery, ear infections, eye infections and tonsillitis.

An acute disease has rapid onset and usually runs a short course, compared to a chronic disease, which has a slow onset and lasts for a long period of time. A chronic disease takes a long time to invade the body, maybe years.

Acute diseases are a natural cleansing of the body. They are trying to purify and cleanse the germs, toxins and foreign material from the system. They need to be treated naturally to prevent the building up for a chronic condition later in life.

The Five Stages of Disease

The first stage of a disease's onset is *incubation*. This is the stage where the inner body is accumulating toxins, poisons, drugs, toxic metals, pesticides and inviting germs, viruses to accumulate. This is the period when the vitality and energy of the body is low. The body feels the stress. The immune system is at its lowest and vitality reserve is low and cannot fight off the invading germs and viruses. When you go and get cold and cough remedies at the drug store, they do sometimes relieve the coughs, runny nose and congestion, but do so by stopping the natural cleansing process. This throws back into the system the toxins which nature was attempting to eliminate. When you add drugs, you are only adding more poisons to the body.

The second stage of a disease is *aggravation*. This is when the immune system is trying to eliminate the toxins, germs, and viruses or whatever is attacking the body. If the immune system is at a low ebb, the disease gradually progresses and can develop into fever and congestion, another way nature is trying to take care of you. This is the stage when symptoms appear and you realize that you are coming down with something.

When you stop the cleansing process in the incubation and aggravation stages the toxins and mucus are thrown further into the organs of the body and will build up in the joints, the lymphatic system and around the heart, and start to "set the soil" for any chronic conditions of those organs.

The third stage is *destruction*. This is the stage where the body is trying to fight the invading germs, viruses or bacteria. This is considered the peak of the crisis. The body is breaking down tissue and old cells are being eliminated. Excess waste is being eliminated along with the buildup chemicals. The body is cleansing itself of those toxic materials before they harden and become difficult to remove. This is the stage where we need to let nature clean at its own pace. When the destruction stage of an acute disease is suppressed, the organs remain permanently damaged. This is the stage where there is a lot of pus and mucus in the body, and the tissues are being broken down. The organs at this stage are holding all this mucus, toxins and pus. What happens to all this pus and mucus when the disease is suppressed by drugs and eating, which stops the cleansing process? The pus stays in the organs and causes pneumonia, tuberculosis, infantile paralysis, spinal meningitis, asthma, emphysema, bronchitis or other diseases.

The fourth stage is the *abatement* stage. This is the stage where excess waste begins to eliminate. The war is being won by the body, with the right treatment by fasting, using only citrus juices and herbs, getting a lot of rest. The poisons, viruses or any foreign matter in the will be overcome and eliminated.

The abatement stage is considered the cleansing stage. The stomach is absorbing the toxins and is attempting to eliminate them through the kidneys and colon. If elimination is suppressed at this stage, the cleansing process is stopped, and the toxins are thrown back into the body. This is the stage when all the glands are filled up, and we can develop lymphatic congestion, glandular secretions, tumors, cysts, moles and skin diseases. This stage sets the environment for all diseases. We can see how we eventually develop chronic diseases.

The fifth stage is the *reconstruction* stage. This is the time when all the stages have run their course and the affected areas have been cleared of morbid accumulations and obstructions. This is the stage when the work of rebuilding begins. The disease has been more or less destructive to the tissues, blood vessels and organs, which all need to be reconstructed. This is the most vital stage when the injured parts of the body must be regenerated with vitamins, minerals, herbs and supplements.

If the reconstruction stage is interfered with or stopped before it is completed, the toxins will continue to invite germs into that area and the affected parts and/or organs will not be entirely cleansed or to become strong. The body will remain in a weakened state. This will lower the capabilities of the immune system and nervous system. The glands remain full, swell up, then shrink and cannot produce the hormones properly. Consequently, we will have a low hormone output, low lymphatic absorption and the intestinal tract will still be coated, leading to indigestion, anemia and deficiencies which causes malnutrition and imbalances. We have suppressed an acute disease at the stage where we should be restoring the cells, but instead we are building up for a chronic disease, and we can then get what is called an incurable disease. Some of the diseases we are treating are autoimmune diseases, such as lupus, diabetes, cancer, heart diseases, candidiasis, arthritis, herpes, chronic fatigue syndrome, and many others.

Symptoms

- coughing
- runny nose
- chills and fever
- aches and pains
- exhaustion
- sore throat
- headaches
- feeling of depression
- cloudy feeling in the head
- heavily coated tongue
- bad breath

Causes

The main cause of colds, flu and all acute diseases is the accumulation of waste matter in the body which cannot readily be eliminated. The body provides an environment where germs, viruses, and parasites are invited. These scavengers will not invade a clean body because they will have nothing to live on.

Germs and viruses are around us constantly and only invade a body when the immune system is low (usually from overeating, working too hard, not enough rest, pessimistic attitude and constipation).

The waste material and toxins that are being eliminated cause irritation and congestion to the internal membranes. This causes symptoms such as inflammation, catarrhal elimination, sneezing, cough, expectoration, mucus discharges, diarrhea, and constipation.

Exposure to cold weather frequently produces colds. The main reason is the cold closes the pores of the skin, and preventing natural elimination through these channels. The skin is the largest elimination organ of the body. It constantly eliminates toxins by way of sweat, vapor, and gases. When the skin shuts down, it puts a load on the kidneys and colon, making them congested and ultimately leading to a cold. The kidneys and colon need to be kept open and clean to prevent acute diseases.

Natural Treatment

The first line of defense is to open up the bowels. Use enemas, colonics or nature's herbal formulas for the bowels. Stop eating. The stomach is gathering the toxins from the cells and trying to eliminate them through the colon. If you eat, the body stops cleansing to digest the food and this throws the toxins back into the organs to solidify, which causes a build-up for chronic diseases later.

Use herbal formulas for the nerves. The body will heal faster when it is relaxed. The nervine herbs will nourish and strengthen the nervous system, and therefore build up the immune system.

Take this time as an excuse to rest in bed, which is the best thing you can do for your body. Free your mind from all worries, and think only good thoughts. Positive feelings will help heal the body.

Dietary Guidelines

Use herbal teas or herbal blends to open up the kidneys and bowels to allow waste material to eliminate properly. A tea should contain uva ursi, which cleans the kidneys, and buckthorn and senna to clean the colon.

Drink only citrus juices, either fresh or frozen. Use lots of fresh pure water. Fresh lemon or lime juice in warm water with grated fresh ginger will help break up congestion, clean the liver and eliminate toxins. Vegetable broths can be used if the body is low in energy.

One all-around formula for acute diseases contains white pine, which helps the skin to eliminate; bayberry, to eliminate toxic waste; ginger and cloves, to cleanse the lymph glands; willow, to help with fevers and produce perspiration; and capsicum, to carry the herbs where they are needed.

There are herbal formulas that will ease coughs, eliminate mucus from the lungs and help ease congestion, pains, nausea, and sore throat.

Massaging the spine with lobelia or other nervine herbs will help the body to relax. Spinal adjustments will help the flow of energy throughout the entire body, and speed up the healing.

NUTRITIONAL SUPPLEMENTS

Digestive Enzymes help in inflammation in the body. They will help break up undigested proteins in the blood and cells. Viruses have protein coating, so enzymes may help to destroy viruses.

Green Drinks, like a mixture of chlorophyll and wheatgrass juice, will clean the blood and help in elimination of toxins.

Vitamin A and Beta Carotene repair damaged tissues and increase resistance to infections.

Vitamin C with bioflavonoids acts as a natural antihistamine, and helps eliminate the symptoms of colds, flu and acute diseases.

Vitamin E speeds healing and protects the lungs and tissues from damage by environmental toxins.

Minerals are essential for all functions of the body. Selenium and zinc will speed healing. Calcium and magnesium protect against toxins and strengthen the nerves.

Acidophilus destroys putrefactive bacteria in the intestinal tract and aids in digestion of nutrients.

Garlic is a natural antibiotic. Mince and use freely for treating colds and flu. Mix with juices and green drinks when taking.

Essential Fatty Acids are essential for balancing body chemistry. They are found in flaxseed, borage, evening primrose, black currant, and salmon oil.

Interferon protects against viruses. This increases the production of fighting T-cells. The following supplements help stimulate the production of interferon in the body: licorice, astragalus, vitamin C with bioflavonoids, chlorophyll, licorice, dulse, kelp, blue-green algae, ginkgo, milk thistle, pau d'arco, schizandra, Siberian ginseng, suma, echinacea, red raspberry, dong quai, ho-shou-wu, wheatgrass juice and germanium.

FACTS AT A GLANCE

• Colds, flu, fever and coughs are nature's way of cleansing the body. They are acute diseases.

• Frequent colds may indicate a conested colon and liver.

- Bad eating habits, exhaustion and malnutrition can cause an imbalance and a low immune system.
- Acute diseases need to be treated naturally to prevent chronic conditions.
- Acute diseases have five stages of cleansing, and when treated naturally will leave the body clean and rejuvenated.
- Germs and viruses will not invade a clean body.
- Avoid eating and use only herbs, citrus juices, pure water and herbal teas when experiencing a cold or flu.

Section 5

The Circulatory and Lymphatic Systems

The health of nations is more important than the wealth of nations.

WILL DURRANT

The Freeway for Nutrition

The circulatory system consists of the blood, heart, arteries, veins and capillaries. Every cell of the body must receive nutrition, and it is the job of the circulatory system to see that rich, nourishing blood reaches all cells and organs of the body for health and vitality.

The American Heart Association has estimated that every 30 seconds there is a death in the United States caused from cardiovascular diseases. Heart disease is the number-one killer in the United States. It is becoming a natural way to die. They call it death from "natural causes." It is not only a disease of the elderly, but is killing people in their prime of life, suddenly and without warning. The very young are showing signs of hardening of the arteries. It is estimated that over half of Americans are accumulating plaque and toxins in their veins.

One doctor stated in 1941, when heart attacks started increasing in the United States, that "atherosclerosis is a disease and not the inevitable consequence of age, since it appears in the young."

John Harvey Kellogg, M.D., in 1916 stated the following: "Diseases of the heart and blood vessels are a common consequence of an acute accumulation of feces in the colon, probably the result of the excessive absorption of toxins to which such accumulations give rise." Fatty deposits in the blood vessels are mainly caused by a toxic colon. An unhealthy colon causes damage to the blood vessels, as well as the small capillaries.

Before World War II, doctors used to treat circulatory diseases as intestinal toxemia or autointoxication. A common statement used was "every physician should realize that the intestinal toxemia are the most important primary and contributing causes of many disorders and diseases of the human body."

Chinese statistics show that "constipation is one of the most common symptoms in ischemic stroke," so Chinese healers often treat stroke by looking for and treating constipation. Chinese studies of stroke patients show recovery rates as high as 88 percent, suggesting that "Chinese medicine is of significance not only in preventing the occurrence of [stroke] but also in treating it." (Keji and S. Jun, "Progress of Research on Ischemic Stroke Treated with Chinese Medicine," *Journal of Traditional Chinese Medicine* 12 [992]: pp 204-10).

The lymphatic system is a part of our immune system and detoxification center. It has the job of carrying nutrients throughout the body as well as removing waste material from all the tissues. The lymphatic fluid has the ability to go deeply into the tissues where blood cannot penetrate, and pick up toxic material in the form of acids and catarrh that has to be eliminated for our protection. These toxins are then passed through the eliminative channels of the lymph glands. These lymph glands or nodes collect the waste material and dump them in the bloodstream. They are then transported to the colon, kidneys, lungs or skin to be eliminated.

The lymph is a clear fluid which bathes all tissues of the body. The vessels that carry this lymph also carry lymphocytes. They act like complex miniature computers, being able to recognize foreign matter, and producing antibodies to combat them. When the body is supplied with proper nutrition, these antibodies destroy poisons before they can cause serious damage and health problems.

The tonsils and appendix are two of the organs that protect the lymph system from becoming overloaded. The tonsils help in the throat area. The toxic material that is eliminated through the tonsils is usually swallowed and with the help of the lymph fluid is reabsorbed into the system and then carried out through the bowels. If the tonsils have been removed, this protection is gone and any infection that enters the mouth goes directly into the lymphatic system, which can cause an overload for the lymph glands to eliminate.

Exercise is very important for the lymphatic system. It needs a pumping action to fulfill its job. The up and down movement on a mini-trampoline causes the lymph vessels to expand and compress, to stretch and relax. This is an action that the lymph fluids need to do their vital job, and eliminate wastes and toxins.

Anemia

Anemia is described as "a disorder characterized by a decrease in hemoglobin in the blood to levels below the normal range, decreased red cell production or increased red cell destruction, or blood loss" (*Mosby's Medical, Nursing, & Allied Health Dictionary*). There are several kinds of anemia. The most common is iron deficiency anemia. There is also folic acid and B12 anemia. More common in African Americans are copper deficiency anemia and sickle cell anemia.

SYMPTOMS

• fatigue
• loss of appetite
• irritability
• general weakness
• pale skin and fingernails
• headaches

CAUSES

Excessive bleeding and malnutrition are two main causes of anemia. Ailments such as hemorrhoids or ulcers, diverticular disease, liver damage, infections, thyroid problems, surgery, and heavy menstrual bleeding and repeated pregnancies can contribute to anemia. Infants and young children on a milk diet, without minerals and essential fatty acids, are prone to anemia.

One of the main causes of anemia is the decreasing ability to assimilate iron and other minerals as we age. Scientific experiments have found that in fatal cases of pernicious anemia, a large amount of iron was driven out of the blood circulation and had settled in the spleen. This revealed that iron was not in short supply but was not being utilized. The importance of making sure there is enough hydrochloric acid in the body for assimilating minerals is vital. An imbalanced diet, poor digestion and wrong food combining add up to poor blood and anemia.

NATURAL TREATMENT

Use herbal therapies to tone up the glands, the circulatory system and the digestive tract. Use blood purifiers; the blood transports nutrients, hormones, electrolytes and waste material to and from every cell in the body. An imbalance or lack of nutrients leads to many problems and symptoms. Healthy blood is the lifeline to all the organs of the body.

DIETARY GUIDELINES

Foods rich in iron are green leafy vegetables, dried apricots, blackstrap molasses, raw egg yolks, dried beans and peas, soy beans and prune juice. Whole grains such as millet and buckwheat, blackberries, cherries, peaches, raisins, sunflower seeds, sesame seeds, egg yolks, fish, sprouts, beets, yams, sweet potatoes, squash, plums, potatoes (with skins) and red cabbage are all rich in nutrition. Fresh green salads will nourish and feed the blood. Vitamin C enhances the absorption of iron. Antacids will decrease iron absorption. Aspirin and many other drugs increase bleeding and can cause anemia. Calcium taken at the same time as iron supplements may inhibit its absorption. Avoid coffee, black or green tea, white flour products, fried foods, excess fats and starches, excess protein, refined sugar, preservatives and additives, canned foods and pasteurized milk.

NUTRITIONAL SUPPLEMENTS

Iron, protein, copper, folic acid and vitamins B6, B12, and C are all essential for the formation of red blood cells.
Vitamin E is needed to help maintain the health of the red blood cells. It helps carry oxygen to the cells.
Vitamins A and B complex aid in the assimilation of iron.
Key herbs include: yellow dock (40 percent iron), dandelion (helps the liver assimilate iron), alfalfa, kelp, dong quai, watercress, barberry, black walnut, burdock, cayenne, echinacea, garlic, gentian, ginger, goldenseal, hawthorn, lobelia, red clover and sarsaparilla.

Bruising

A bruise is an injury involving the rupture of small blood vessels and discoloration without a break in the overlying skin. Most bruises are not serious. You can fall or bump yourself and a bruise is the result.

SYMPTOMS

- ruptured skin capillaries (marked by discoloration of blood)
- black and blue patches

CAUSES

In rare cases, a bruise is a sign of problems elsewhere in the body. It could be kidney and liver disorders. Anemia can cause bruising as well as blood disorders and allergies. Purplish bumps under the skin that do not heal and look like bruises could be a symptom of AIDS.

Lack of proper nutrition such as a vitamin and mineral deficiency can be a factor. Drugs such as aspirin and anti-clotting medications can cause bruising. Bruises can also be a sign of cancer.

NATURAL TREATMENT

Strengthen the blood and vessels by eating a diet rich in dark green leafy vegetables, steamed and raw vegetables, and juices containing carrot, celery, parsley and wheatgrass. Chlorophyll will build and purify the blood. Eliminating acid foods and adding alkaline foods will clean the blood. Herbs to help in bruising are alfalfa, bee pollen, black walnut, burdock, aloe vera, cayenne, horsetail, kelp, pau d'arco and white oak bark.

NUTRITIONAL SUPPLEMENTS

Vitamins A and D are healing.
B-complex with extra B12 and folic acid can help.
Vitamin C with bioflavonoids strengthens the vessels to prevent bruises.
Iron supplements are beneficial; those containing yellow dock assimilate easier.
Zinc is very healing.
Calcium and magnesium are beneficial.
Blue-green algae nourishes the blood.
Lecithin is essential for healthy veins.
Essential Fatty Acids play an important role in healthy blood.

FACTS AT A GLANCE

• Anemia and bruising are nutritionally-based disorders.
• Eat a diet high in leafy green vegetables and fresh foods.
• Key supplements can help build the blood and strengthen the blood vessels.
• Healthy blood is the lifeline to all organs of the body.

Arteriosclerosis and High Blood Pressure

Every year, over three times as many Americans die from cardiovascular diseases as were lost in combat during the entirety of World War II. Arteriosclerosis is a generic term describing the thickening, loss of elasticity and calcification of arterial walls. This causes decreased blood supply to the brain, among other problems. Very simply, arteriosclerosis is the presence of fatty deposits in the arteries, which have the tendency to restrict free flow of blood. This can cause hypertension or high blood pressure. This is considered to be a "silent killer." Hypertension causes the heart to overwork and can lead to serious diseases such as blindness from retinal hemorrhage, heart or kidney damage, or even stroke.

Symptoms

Hypertension is called a "silent killer" because its symptoms are hard to detect. Two in five people do not even know they have the disorder and four out of five with hypertension are either unaware or not in control of their condition. It is essential to have blood pressure check-ups often. It does not cause symptoms of anxiety, heart poundings, increase in pulse rate or similar symptoms of other diseases

Causes

As fine capillaries become more and more clogged, additional energy is demanded to maintain balanced blood circulation. It's as if freeway rush-hour traffic were expected to move freely down an alley too narrow for a Cadillac. Then with the thickening of the blood which comes from the waste products of protein and starch metabolism (mucus), resistance against the blood flow becomes greater. This requires increased energy for circulation, thereby putting added strain not only upon the arteries, but the heart itself. Excess sodium in the system raises blood pressure. The average American consumes about thirty times the body's need for sodium. Research shows that most people with high blood pressure lack adequate calcium in their diet.

Natural Treatment

Julian M. Whitaker, M.D., in his book, *Reversing Heart Disease,* says, "Voluminous research shows that dietary changes could eliminate high blood pressure in many hypertensive patients. In spite of that, the routine approach for many M.D.s is to immediately start a patient on drugs before, and usually without any recommendation for a dietary change. The dangerous side effects of the drugs used make this approach, in my opinion, often more harmful to the patient than beneficial." Regular exercise helps to improve blood flow and helps prevent the accumulation of plaque on blood vessel walls. Walking, bicycling and other similar types of outdoor exercise are good examples. The elimination of all mental stress and worries, as well as environmental sources of metal poisoning are also vital. Smoking is a definite "no-no," for this habit constricts the arteries and aggravates the condition further.

Dietary Guidelines

An herbal salt substitute is a wonderful way to cut down on salt and yet have tasty food. Kelp and dulse are also very good as salt substitutes. An herbal calcium supplement containing herbs like comfrey, alfalfa, oatstraw and horsetail is an excellent way to increase necessary calcium and other minerals essential for a healthy body. Many health-oriented doctors are finding that using herbs and changing the diet has eliminated high blood pressure in many people. Even though the following story is of one man's experience, the program would work equally well for a woman. In the book, *Helping Yourself with Natural Remedies,* Terry Willard, Ph.D,. tells of a man with blood pressure of 180/120. This man started taking one capsule of cayenne pepper during meals, one garlic/parsley capsule twice daily, one liver formula twice daily, 2,000 mg of vitamin C (with 1,000 mg of bioflavonoids), and 200 I.U. of vitamin E. His diet excluded all dairy and white flour products, salt, fried foods and preservatives. He ate lots of whole grains and raw vegetables. In three months it was 135/90, at which time he slowly lowered his therapy. A raw food diet of fruits, vegetables, seeds, nuts and sprouts exerts a powerful protective action against arteriosclerosis. Short juice fasts, the eating of several small meals rather than two or three large ones, eating in moderation and the elimination of meat, salt, white sugar, white flour and all refined and processed foods are also important.

NUTRITIONAL SUPPLEMENTS

Butcher's Broom has a toning effect on the internal surface of the veins. It protects against strokes, hemorrhoids, varicose veins and other circulatory problems. It prevents the post-operative tendency towards circulatory complications like blood clots.

Bugleweed acts like digitalis in calming the pulse, and is excellent for heart diseases whenever irregular heartbeat is involved.

Capsicum or Cayenne stops bleeding and helps prevent heart attacks and stroke.

Garlic dissolves built-up cholesterol and loosens it out of the arteries. It builds the immune system and stimulates the lymphatic system.

Hawthorn Berry nourishes the heart and helps the circulation. It helps prevent hardening of the arteries, regulates blood pressure, and helps strengthen the nerves.

Gotu Kola relieves high blood pressure, mental fatigue and senility.

Ginkgo biloba has been shown inh European studies to increase blood flow in the brain, which improves memory. It also helps prevent and treat stokes by preventing the formation of blood clots. This herb helps nourish the arteries and relieves pain, cramping and weakness. It increases circulation of blood flow in the retina and prevents macular degeneration. Ear problems are improved with ginkgo, due to improved blood flow to the nerves of the inner ear. It increases oxygen and blood flow to the extremities, improves mental clarity and inhibits free radical scavengers from destroying cells. It supplies nutritional support to all areas of the body. It dilates the blood vessels, allowing improved blood flow to the tissues. It eliminates waste material and inhibits the abnormal clumping of blood platelets which can contribute to heart problems, strokes and artery conditions.

Co Q-10 increases strength of the heart, relieves angina, protects against heart attacks, lowers high blood pressure, and nourishes the immune system.

Essential Fatty Acids improve gland and enzyme function and help control blood clotting and arterial spasms. They balance cholesterol and triglyceride levels.

Vitamin E is a natural antioxidant. It helps prevent blood-clot formation. Vitamin E dilates the capillaries, enabling blood to flow more freely into the muscle tissues. It strengthens the heart and improves overall circulation.

FACTS AT A GLANCE

• High blood pressure is considered to be a "silent killer."
• It is essential to have regular blood pressure check-ups.
• Eating a diet high in fresh foods will promote optimal cardiovascular health.
• Exercising regularly will strengthen the heart.

Varicose Veins and Hemorrhoids

Vein varicosity is considered to be a major circulatory disorder in this modern age. Varicose veins and hemorrhoids are caused from chronic constipation and circulatory system weakness. Liver congestion has been implicated as another cause. Varicose veins occur most often in the legs. Weakness in the veins allows blood to accumulate and stretch the capillaries and veins and cause discoloring, tenderness and sometimes pain.

SYMPTOMS

• blue, bulging veins on the legs
• pain and swelling of veins
• leg cramps
• heavy feeling in the legs

• tired legs
• dull aches and pains in the legs

There are external hemorrhoids and internal hemorrhoids. External ones are easily identifiable and are usually more painful. Internal hemorrhoids may be present for years and not cause trouble. They can also appear externally if they become swollen and protrude the anal ring. Bleeding may be the first sign of internal hemorrhoids. Constant bleeding over a period of time can cause anemia.

CAUSES

Varicose veins and hemorrhoids are commonly associated with pregnancy, junk food diet (clogs the circulatory system), lack of exercise, sitting while working, heavy lifting, and obesity. It is found in those who consume low-fiber diets. If left untreated, varicose veins can lead to phlebitis, leg ulcers, permanently swollen legs, pulmonary emboli (or clots in the lungs), and even surface leg hemorrhaging.

NATURAL TREATMENT

Blood purification herbs, circulatory strengthening and lower bowel cleansers will help in varicose veins and hemorrhoids. Liver cleansing will promote better filtering of toxins.

Exercise will help strengthen the veins and increase circulation. Just walking will help. It will help prevent deposits of clotting blood within the veins. Don't cross your legs while sitting. Jogging, cycling, and hiking will help prevent the tendency toward varicose veins. A "bone, flesh and cartilage" herbal salve on a raw red potato piece or clove of garlic can be used as a natural suppository for hemorrhoids. Use several times a week. Sitz baths, when continued for several days, will help strengthen the veins. The sitz bath involves using two basins, one with hot water, and one cold. Use the hot basin first and cold last. The warm water relaxes the spasms of the muscles and the cold one tightens the tissues.

DIETARY GUIDELINES

Eat a high-fiber diet, using whole grains, fresh salads, and vegetables (containing minerals for strengthening the veins). Figs, raisins and prunes, soaked in pure water before use, are nourishing. Citrus fruit, especially the white inner skin of the rind, will strengthen and heal the veins with its high bioflavonoid content. Oat bran is very beneficial for keeping the veins clean. Buckwheat contains rutin, a bioflavonoid which strengthens the veins and decreases the tendency of the capillaries to break easily. Use sprouted seeds and grains and fresh fruits. Chewing food well and correct food combining will help assimilate and eliminate food properly. Use short fasts, using juices made from green vegetables, chlorophyll and pure water. Carrot and celery juices are also beneficial. Avoid margarine (it clogs the veins), and all unnatural fats. Eat meat, such as chicken and fish, sparingly, and avoid pork and red meat. Sugar and white-flour foods (candy, cookies, ice cream, and pastries) will clog the veins. Sugar leeches the calcium from the body. One of the first places calcium and minerals are taken from the body are the veins. This can cause varicose veins and may develop into phlebitis.

NUTRITIONAL SUPPLEMENTS

Vitamin A strengthens the veins.

Vitamin C with bioflavonoids strengthens the veins and capillaries.

Vitamin E is a vital nutrient for varicose veins, and protects the cells and blood vessel walls from damage.

B-complex, Silicon, Selenium, Zinc, Calcium and Vitamin D are also very important in healing veins.

Key herbs include: aloe vera, black walnut (rich in minerals), butcher's broom (strengthens the blood vessels and keeps them clean), capsicum, cascara sagrada (colon rebuilder), comfrey, goldenseal, horsetail (contains silicon), kelp (strengthens and cleans veins), mullein oil (applied externally relieves pain), oatstraw, pau d'arco, white oak bark (strengthens veins), and witch hazel (external). Other vital herbs include alfalfa, bayberry, buckthorn, lobelia, parsley, red raspberry, slippery elm, uva ursi and wood betony.

Other nutritional supplements include bee pollen, blue-green algae, psyllium, spirulina (blue-green algae), salmon oil, germanium and Co Q-10. Calendula (marigold) ointment helps in itching and pain. External applications include oak bark poultice, comfrey and goldenseal ointment, and clay packs.

FACTS AT A GLANCE

• Exercise will help strengthen the veins and increase circulatory flow.
• Use supplements that nourish the circulatory system.
• Eating a high-fiber diet will inhibit occurrence of varicose veins.
• Some women have a habit of crossing their legs while sitting. This can contribute to varicose veins by putting a strain on blood vessel walls. Make a conscious effort to sit with your spine and hips aligned.

Section 6

The Glandular System

Look to your health; and if you have it, praise God, and value it next to a good conscience; for health is the second blessing that we mortals are capable of; a blessing that money cannot buy.

IZAAK WALTON

The Body's Balancing Act

The glandular system has many important functions necessary for health and well-being. The endocrine glands secrete hormones for activities of the body directly into the bloodstream. The glands get their orders directly from the brain and spinal cord and have life and death control over the entire body. It is essential that we keep these glands healthy with the finest nutrition possible. It is important and vital that the bloodstream be pure and that the veins and arteries be clear and free of fatty deposits. The blood must be flowing freely and the heart functioning normally to get pure blood to all the glandular areas at all times if we expect excellent mental and physical health.

Scientists used to believe that the brain was insulated from the rest of the body by the blood/brain barrier, and that diet did not have much to do with a healthy endocrine system. A major breakthrough occurred when Dr. Richard J. Wurtman and his colleagues at the Massachusetts Institute of Technology demonstrated that diet does contain precursors of brain neurotransmitters which modulate aspects of mood, mind, memory and behavior.

Dr. Wurtman has demonstrated in his research that carbohydrates in a meal stimulate the production of insulin which, in turn, facilitates the uptake of the amino acid tryptophan which is then used by specific regions of the brain for the synthesis and secretion of the neurotransmitter serotonin, which has a calming effect upon mood.

We know that an iodine deficiency has an impact on the thyroid and can produce goiter. Zinc deficiency may have an adverse impact upon thymus secretion of the hormone thymosin which, in turn, has a T-lymphocyte regulatory effect.

Nutrition also has an impact upon the behavior mechanisms of the hypothalamus and pituitary. Animal studies over the years have shown that marginal deprivation of certain nutrients and calories can result in suppression of normal appetite mechanisms in the hypothalamus, resulting in eating disorders. This may shed a new light on eating disorders such as anorexia nervosa, bulimia and compulsive eating, and the effect lack of nutrients has on the endocrine and nervous systems.

Proper nutrition does have an impact on a healthy endocrine system. Each gland plays an important role to the overall health of the body. When one gland isn't working properly, it can affect other glands. It is important that we understand the glands, and the nutrients that will clean, build and strengthen them.

THE GLANDULAR SYSTEM AND RAW FOOD

Raw foods are necessary for the glandular system. Cooked food kills the enzymes and causes the endocrine glands to become overworked which leads to body intoxication and diseases such as hypoglycemia, diabetes and obesity. Cooked foods overstimulate the glands and cause the body to retain excess weight. The enzymes from live food help the body to maintain proper metabolism.

The problem arises when the glands do not receive the nutrients necessary to satisfy the body's needs. When this happens, the glands overstimulate the digestive organs and demand more food (because the body is not nutritionally satisfied). This produces an over-secretion of hormones and an unhealthy appetite, which finally results in exhaustion of the hormone-producing glands.

Glandular Function

The glandular system consists of the pituitary gland, thyroid gland, parathyroid gland, thymus gland, pineal gland, the testes, ovaries, pancreas, hypothalamus and adrenal glands.

The glands work together in producing and excreting chemical substances known as hormones. The hormones are responsible for coordinating and controlling various organs and tissues so the body works smoothly and efficiently. The hormones are released into the bloodstream. The hypothalamus, located at the base of the brain, regulates the network of glands along with the nervous system and the pituitary gland. When disorders of the endocrine system develop, they usually consist of either underactivity or overactivity of one or more glands. An imbalance is usually created by the lack of nutrients to the glands.

THE ADRENALS

The adrenals protect us from stress. Aching joints are one sign that the adrenals are exhausted, too exhausted to produce the hormones that prevent pain and inflammation. Healthy adrenals improve digestion, burn fat more efficiently and give the body strength throughout the day. Herbs which help in a crisis situation for the adrenals are lobelia and cayenne. Additional herbs for the adrenals are licorice, hawthorn, chamomile, skullcap, rose hips, and ginseng. The adrenals also benefit from vitamins A, C, B-complex and pantothenic acid.

THE THYMUS GLAND

The thymus gland is considered the youth gland. It helps remove "negative charges" from the body. It helps create an attitude of positive thoughts and feelings. The thymus needs beta-carotene, B-complex, and zinc. It especially needs calcium and phosphorus. Nervine herbs like lobelia, hops, passion flower, and skullcap are beneficial.

THE PINEAL GLAND

The pineal gland puts us at peace with ourselves. It needs stimulation from electromagnetic impulses from the optic nerves. Sunlight entering the eyes triggers retinal nerve impulses which travel to the pineal gland. The nerve impulses from the pineal gland are fed to the hypothalamus and pituitary, which affect many of the vital functions of the body.

THE PITUITARY GLAND

The pituitary is the "master gland," acting as a synergist to most all of the glandular extracts. The pituitary, when healthy, protects us from fatigue due to excessive mental stress. Those who cannot tolerate stress and cannot work under pressure need the pituitary gland strengthened. Vitamins B6, E, and B-complex are needed, as well as manganese, selenium, trace minerals, and amino acids ornithine, tryptophan, and taurine. Herbs that help the pituitary are kelp (helps all the glands), gotu kola, and ginseng.

THE PANCREAS

The pancreas is important in the digestion of food, the secretion of insulin for the maintenance of proper blood-sugar levels and for activating enzyme processes in the body. Nutrients for the pituitary are B-complex, chromium, selenium, manganese and sodium, and the amino acids isoleucine and leucine. Herbs that help are alfalfa, juniper berries, uva ursi, saw palmetto, goldenseal and ho shou wu.

THE THYROID GLAND

The thyroid gland secretes a hormone called thyroxine which regulates the rate of metabolism of human cells. Hyperthyroidism occurs when an excess of the thyroid hormone creates more heat in the body, thereby burning more calories and losing more weight, in spite of a healthy appetite.

Hypothyroidism exists when there is insufficient thyroid hormone. The body tends to feel cold and the individual becomes puffy-faced, obese, sluggish and dull-witted. B-complex vitamins and the minerals iodine, potassium, sodium, and the amino acid tyrosine are especially needed. Herbs which help include kelp, black walnut, white oak bark and gentian.

Premenstrual Syndrome (PMS)

Premenstrual syndrome is not the silent malady it once was. Women used to receive indifference when they exposed their feelings and fears about what was going on in their bodies and minds. They were usually told that it was all in their heads. The doctors listened to the complaints of women but could not understand or recognize the symptoms and didn't know the treatments, so they thought that PMS was incurable. They would tell the women to go home to bed and take an aspirin, or for more serious cases they wrote millions of prescriptions for tranquilizers.

Symptoms of PMS

• pelvic pain
• irritability
• lethargy
• bloating
• depression
• impatience
• nervousness
• swelling of breasts

There are at least one hundred and fifty symptoms associated with PMS. For some women, the pain is severe, tension builds up, and migraine headaches and mood swings are so severe that they lead to violence. When a condition becomes so debilitating that lawyers can use PMS successfully as a mitigating circumstance in defending women accused of crimes, then something must be done. It has been used as an excuse for murder, suicide, child beating and car accidents. It disrupts growing families, husband and wife relationships, and efficiency in the workplace.

CAUSES

Hormonal Imbalance: Tests have shown that the flow of estrogen through the liver can be regulated by providing B-complex vitamins in the diet. When excess estrogen builds up and the liver is unable to detoxify it, there is havoc created in the body — from water retention to severe mental anguish. Excess estrogen has a strong effect on women in various ways. Changes in hormonal levels are noticeable anywhere from four days to two weeks before the period begins. Definite drops in the pituitary and ovarian hormones have been measured, which may be the reason for the emotional reaction during this time.

Malnutrition and Constipation: This occurs when nutrients are not being properly assimilated into the bloodstream. Blood is the life of the body and it needs to be kept clean and pure so it can carry nutrients to the system and carry off all waste material. Constipation puts pressure on the uterus and causes pain.

Stress: We are confronted with all kinds of stress in our modern world. It affects the immune system and depletes nutrients from the body. We need to replace nutrients so we can properly handle stress.

Calcium Depletion: Blood calcium drops days prior to menstruation. It occurs when ovaries are least active and continues steadily until even after the onset of bleeding. Steady calcium decrease causes tension, headaches, nervousness, insomnia and depression. The body needs adequate calcium, vitamin D and magnesium.

Hypoglycemia and other ailments: Hypoglycemia can increase the severity of PMS by affecting the immune system. Many women have experienced allergies, food or chemical sensitivities, migraine headaches, flu and other illness just before their period when their immunity level is down.

NATURAL TREATMENT

Although PMS is not a disease nor a neurosis, it has the symptoms of both. Some doctors consider it a monthly endocrine disorder, and feel that it is essential to feed and stimulate the glands, as well as the circulatory, nervous and digestive systems with proper nutrients. Change the diet and clean the bowels before menstruation. Herbal laxatives are very useful. They rebuild the bowels and provide proper function for the whole system.

Vitamins A and C should be used daily. The nervine herbs will build and feed the nervous system. The body craves and demands food to nourish it and if it isn't satisfied, this puts more stress upon the body. This can cause irritability and emotional problems as well as disease.

DIETARY GUIDELINES

A hypoglycemia diet has been used successfully to help PMS. This is where you keep the blood sugar levels balanced by eating six small meals a day, rather than three large ones. A diet consisting of foods such as unprocessed nuts, seeds, chicken, fish, grains, beans, split peas, lentils, green leafy vegetables and raw fruits is recommended. Avoid coffee, chocolate, sugar, salt and alcohol. They increase irritability and interfere with the metabolism of nutrients to the body.

NUTRITIONAL SUPPLEMENTS

Vitamin A helps to regulate the cycle and nourishes the glands. It helps alleviate monthly skin problems, protects the body from disease, and rebuilds the cells.

B-Complex Vitamins are essential to combat fatigue, help reduce sugar cravings, and weight fluctuation and bloating. B-complex vitamins are necessary to assist the liver in detoxifying excess estrogen in the body and preventing hormonal imbalance. B2 is needed during stress. A lack of it can cause depression, hysteria, trembling and fatigue. B6 helps in treating tension, aggression, depression and irritability. It also acts as a natural diuretic. It restores the balance between progesterone and estrogen. Daily supplements of 40 to 100 mg have been used successfully. B12 deficiency can cause depression, fatigue, loss of appetite and irritability. It is needed daily.

Calcium and Magnesium deficiencies can cause headaches, nervous symptoms and fluid retention. These nutrients relieve cramps and nervousness. They prevent cramps in the uterine wall and leg muscles, and also prevent also irritability and depression. Magnesium suppresses the craving for chocolate and increases the absorption of B-vitamins.

Vitamin C with bioflavonoids repairs cells, relieves stress, and builds the immune system. It helps regulate the menstrual flow when it is too heavy. The bioflavonoids also help with menstrual regularity.

Alfalfa helps the body digest food and supplements. It is rich in vitamins, minerals (especially calcium and magnesium) and enzymes.

Black Cohosh contains "plant hormones" known as phytosterols. These estrogenic-like properties help in delayed menstrual flow, cramping, and menopause. It contains potassium and magnesium, which act as nerve sedatives. It has a built-in "safety valve" because it will cause a headache if a person takes too much.

Chamomile soothes the nerves and relieves stomach cramps. It is very useful for menstrual cramps. This herb contains high amounts of calcium and magnesium, as well as tryptophan, which acts as a sedative.

Dong Quai is a Chinese herb that helps to balance hormones in the body. It is suggested that it be taken at least five days before the onset of menstruation, before the body reaches its estrogen-progesterone low. It nourishes and strengthens the nerves and reproductive organs.

Cat's Claw is an herb that has been shown to help with irregularities of the female cycle. It also detoxifies the intestinal tract.

Evening Primrose Oil is rich in gamma-linolenic acid (GLA). GLA is essential for the body's synthesis of prostaglandins, hormone-like compounds that control many body processes. Evening primrose oil helps minimize PMS symptoms.

Vitamin E helps to ease the symptoms of PMS. It relieves pain, helps reduce cramps, increases blood circulation, and inhibits breast tenderness. Vitamin E is important for the body's production of sex hormones.

Iodine nourishes the thyroid gland. The thyroid gland produces the hormone thyroxine, which is necessary for the breakdown of estrogen. Too little thyroxine means too much estrogen. This can promote intense and poorly timed menstrual periods, water retention and even blood clotting. Kelp is an herb high in natural iodine, as well as many other minerals, and helps regulate the iodine the body needs.

Vitex agnus-castus is a plant native to Greece and Italy. It helps normalize the menstrual cycle and flow. It assists the body's elimination of excessive estrogen, and alleviates premenstrual syndrome symptoms. It also helps with teenage acne. Vitex balances all the female hormones. It is believed to work by regulating the actions of the pituitary gland, the master gland of the body.

Wild Yam Cream has helped with the estrogen/progesterone balance in the body when applied topically.

FACTS AT A GLANCE

* PMS can be treated nutritionally.
* PMS is not a disease nor a neurosis.
* PMS is caused by too much estrogen in the body.
* Cleansing the blood, liver and bowels with key supplements helps balance hormone levels.

Cysts and Tumors

A cyst is a closed sac or pouch with a definite wall which contains fluid, semifluid or solid material. A ganglion is a cyst full of a jelly-like material, occurring in association with joints and tendons. They are common on the back of the hand, wrist or foot, sometimes occurring by the elbow or other joints. A tumor, on the other hand, is a spontaneous growth of tissue that forms an abnormal mass which performs no physiological function.

SYMPTOMS

There are benign tumors and malignant tumors. Benign tumors are usually limited in growth, are isolated and can occur anywhere in the body. Fibroids are benign tumors that are often found in the uterus. Thousands of hysterectomies are performed each year because of the presence of fibroid tumors in the uterus. Fibroid tumors and fibrocystic breast disease are caused by excessive estrogen in the body. They can be prevented and eliminated by detoxifying the body through the liver and intestinal tract.

Fibrocystic breast disease involves over fifty percent of adult females in the United States. This is a benign lump condition which rarely turns cancerous. It is believed that the problem stems from too much estrogen that the liver cannot filter because of congestion in the colon. This bad estrogen is responsible for proliferating tissue where it travels to the primary estrogen receptors of the body (especially the breasts and uterus), which causes cysts and growths. Excessive estradiol, as well as other toxins, back up into the bloodstream and enter the breasts, brain or other parts of the body to cause lumps, congestion or other diseases in the system. When the liver is congested, it cannot filter harmful substances such as caffeine, found in coffee, tea, soda and chocolate.

Endometriosis is a rather common disease in our present age. It is estimated that 40 to 60 percent of women who undergo hysterectomies have endometriosis. It is an outgrowth of the uterine lining into the pelvic cavity. It can cause irregular bleeding, pain during intercourse and menses, severe pelvic pain and even infertility. (For more information, please see the "Estrogen" section).

Malignant tumors are cancerous and can spread to other parts of the body. Even when surgically removed, malignant tumors tend to recur after surgery. It seems logical that the blood and lymphatic system have the ability to spread cancer cells to any weakened part of the body.

Blocked energy in the body as well as toxic blood, excessive mucus and undigested food can promote growths such as lumps, cysts and tumors. Herbal therapy and a diet change have proven very effective for many people.

CAUSES

One cause of cyst and tumor growth is the lack of potassium in the diet. In the 1920s, Dr. Otto Warburn, a Nobel prize winner, demonstrated that the metabolism (chemical changes incidental to life and growth) of cancerous tissue differs radically from that of normal tissue. Normal tissue acquires its nourishment from oxidation and usually dies if deprived of oxygen. But cancerous tissue subsists by a process in which cell-nutritive substances are broken down by specialized chemicals, much as food is broken down in ordinary digestion, and so needs little or no oxygen to exist. Experiments have established that normal animal tissue may become cancerous if deprived of oxygen for long intervals. It is the blood that provides the cells of the body with oxygen, so the condition of the bloodstream determines cancer development. Wherever the blood supply is poor — such as around or near scars, ulcers, in atrophied organs, injuries or any place where energy is blocked — malignant tumors can develop.

NATURAL TREATMENT

Short fasts and a diet rich in potassium foods such as almonds, apples, dried apricots, bananas, beans, beets, broccoli, carrots, dulse, figs, goat milk, grapes, kale, olives, parsley, pecans, rice bran, sunflower seeds, watercress and wheat bran and germ are very beneficial in eliminating cysts and tumors.

Potassium-rich foods and herbs increase alkalinity and eliminate acid in the body. Potassium is vital to help neutralize acids and toxins. Potassium reduces excessive gastric acidity and intestinal acidity and promotes good peristalsis of the stomach and intestines. Potassium prevents ailments and promotes good health.

Nutritional Supplements

Coenzyme Q-10 promotes immune function and carries oxygen to the cells.

Garlic has been shown to reduce tumors. It is a natural antibiotic that acts on germs and viruses.

Vitamin C cleans the veins, promotes a healthy immune system, and helps prevent diseases.

Digestive Enzymes aid in the breakdown of undigested foods to help prevent stagnation. They also strengthen the immune system.

Kelp supplies essential minerals, cleans the veins, and promotes a strong immune system.

Echinacea is the "king" of cleansers. It is a great blood cleaner and helps protect the lymphatic system. It also purifies the blood.

Suma, Ginkgo biloba and Gotu Kola promote a healthy immune system and increase circulation. Blocked circulation is the beginning of many health problems, including cysts and tumors.

Lecithin helps to regulate metabolism and breakdown fat and cholesterol. It prevents plaque from adhering to artery walls. Lecithin slows down the aging process and aids in rebuilding brain cells.

Psyllium fiber prevents stagnation in the colon and the blood.

Vitex agnus-castus has been known to help with some types of uterine cysts (fibroids) and has been used to treat endometriosis. Blood purifying herbal combinations which contain herbs like burdock, goldenseal, echinacea, and red clover help clean the entire system, as well as the cells. It will purify the blood and provide minerals to strengthen and heal the body. These herbs kill toxins, germs, nourish the pituitary gland, loosen mucus from the lungs, dissolve hardened mucus (as in cysts and tumors), kill infections, strengthen the adrenals, dissolve cholesterol, and improve liver function. (For more information, on this topic, please refer to the chapter on Estrogen).

Facts at a Glance

- Fibroid tumors, fibrocystic breast disease, and endometriosis are caused by excessive estrogen production in the body.

- Another cause of cysts and tumor growth is the lack of potassium in the diet.
- Malignant tumors can develop wherever the circulation is inhibited.
- Cancerous tumors thrive in an oxygen-deficient environment.

Diabetes

The pancreas, a small pink gland located below and behind the stomach, is an important organ of the human digestive system. It takes part in the digestion of proteins, starches, sugars and fats, and is the endocrine gland which controls blood sugar.

The small islands of glandular tissue which are scattered throughout the pancreas, called the Islets of Langerhans, produce insulin. If the pancreas cannot secrete enough insulin, the liver will be unable to store the sugar which is so necessary for strengthening the muscles. When the liver can no longer get insulin, the sugar enters the bloodstream, kidneys, and urine, causing diabetes. Diabetes is a disease in which the body cannot utilize all the sugar that enters the bloodstream.

Diabetes is increasing at a fast rate; more than 10 million Americans have this disease. It is estimated that two out of five of them do not realize they have diabetes. Americans eat too many fast foods. Diabetes is unknown in countries where people can't afford to overeat. People with diabetes are up to four times more likely to die from a heart attack, and those with diabetes have a greater risk of having strokes.

SYMPTOMS OF DIABETES

- excessive thirst
- excessive urination
- excessive hunger
- general weakness
- skin disorders that do not heal quickly
- blurred vision
- tingling leg cramps
- dry mouth

Causes

There are two types of diabetes. The first is Type 1, or juvenile diabetes mellitus, also called insulin-dependent diabetes mellitus (IDDM). In this type, the pancreas does not produce insulin, the hormone which delivers glucose to the cells. This is a more serious diabetes and almost always develops in childhood.

In Type 2 diabetes, the pancreas produces insulin but the cells have too few chemical receptors and the cells starve, resulting in a lack of energy. The major cause of type 2 is now thought to be obesity. Overeating and eating the wrong kinds of food are the major causes.

Natural treatment

Many doctors believe that diabetes can be controlled through proper diet. It is also important to keep the bowels well-regulated, and get plenty of rest and sunshine. It is better to eat small, frequent meals than to overeat. Too much food at one time is very hard on the pancreas, and eventually may paralyze its normal activity. Exercise and skin brushing will speed the cleansing and healing. Exercise helps the body use up excess blood sugar. Regular aerobic exercise will benefit the body's blood sugar levels. There is a theory that many cases of diabetes, especially juvenile diabetes, are linked to parasite infestation of the bowels and pancreas. Use blood purifiers, lower bowel cleansers and parasite herbal combinations.

Dietary Guidelines

High-quality natural foods are important: whole grains such as buckwheat, millet, barley, brown rice, and whole oats, and raw vegetables and raw fruits are among the best. Raw foods stimulate the pancreas to increase insulin production. Sprouted grains can be added to salads and in vegetable casseroles. A high-fiber diet helps to lower blood triglycerides in diabetics and prediabetics. Fiber has the ability to repair faulty sugar metabolism by its complex effects on gastrointestinal functioning. Protein foods such as cottage cheese, yogurt, kefir, nuts and avocados are also good. Vegetables such as asparagus, green beans, okra, celery, watercress, parsley, alfalfa, and Jerusalem artichokes are beneficial in a diabetic's diet. Jerusalem artichokes contain a starch that the pancreas can handle.

Sugar is the modern person's weakness and downfall. It is prevalent in our diets, and difficult to avoid. It is found in canned, frozen and fast foods. Read labels and become familiar with the different forms of sugar: i.e., sucrose, dextrose, fructose, high fructose corn syrup, honey, molasses, etc.

Avoid a heavy meat diet, soft drinks, caffeine, tobacco, starches, and all denatured foods, including white sugar and white flour products.

NUTRITIONAL SUPPLEMENTS

Use natural *vitamin A* to help protect the eyes from damage (beta-carotene is difficult for the diabetic to convert into vitamin A). All vitamins are involved directly or indirectly in maintaining normal sugar metabolism.

B-complex Vitamins help to cut down on insulin intake; they also strengthen and repair nerves.

Vitamin C with bioflavonoids is essential for arterial health. It cleans the veins and strengthens the immune system.

Vitamin E is necessary to help the body store sugar as glycogen, and helps reduce artery complications.

The Amino Acids L-carnitine and L-glutamine help the liver to metabolize fat.

Zinc is important. Many diabetics are low in this nutrient and it helps the body manufacture insulin.

Chromium helps the body stabilize blood sugar levels. It is the major mineral involved with insulin production. Some nutritionists believe that many cases of diabetes could actually be a chromium deficiency, induced by eating a lot of refined grains and sugars. This type of diet is very low in chromium.

Cat's Claw (uña de gato) is useful for diabetes and helps the body get rid of parasites. This remarkable herb has anti-inflammatory, antioxidant, and antimicrobial properties.

Goldenseal has the ability to regulate sugar and prevent the body mechanism from flooding the system with too much insulin when certain foods are eaten. It helps the body resist disease and build natural immunity to harmful micro-organisms. It is a natural antibiotic and has the ability to stop internal bleeding and internal swelling; very important for diabetics. Goldenseal contains vitamins A, C and B-complex. It also supplies phosphorus, calcium, potassium, zinc, sulphur and copper.

Juniper is high in natural insulin. It has the ability to restore the pancreas where there has been no permanent damage. It is excellent for combatting infections. It is a natural antibiotic and diuretic. Juniper is high in vitamin C and the trace mineral cobalt.

Uva Ursi contains moderate amounts of natural insulin. It is very helpful for excess sugar in the system.

Comfrey has a healing effect on every organ of the body. It has a soothing and protective effect internally. It coats the lower bowels with a nutritious substance that strengthens as well as heals. Comfrey contains an average of about 28 percent usable protein, which is beneficial for diabetes. It helps establish normal balance in the system. Comfrey is high in calcium and phosphorus. It contains potassium and is rich in vitamins A, C, and E. It contains B12, B1, and B2. It also contains eighteen amino acids.

Dandelion is beneficial in the system as a blood purifier and tonic. It increases the activity of the pancreas, and also helps alleviate congestion in that organ. Dandelion benefits the functions of the liver and stimulates it to detoxify poisons. It is rich in vitamins A and C, as well as potassium, calcium, sodium, and some phosphorus and iron.

FACTS AT A GLANCE

- Keeping the bowels well-regulated will decrease chances of diabetes.
- Plenty of rest allows the digestive organs to function properly.
- Eating small frequent meals allows organs to function properly.
- Eat a nutritious diet and stay away from denatured foods.
- Taking key supplements can help offset any nutritional deficiencies caused by diet.

Hypoglycemia

Many women suffer from low blood sugar, otherwise called hypo-glycemia. Even though it is a physical condition, it causes mental and emotional changes in the body. Many doctors in the medical field claim it does not exist. It does exist and is increasing rapidly, primarily because of poor eating habits. The American diet is strongly imbalanced with refined foods which damage the nervous and immune systems, and initiate the development of hypoglycemia.

Symptoms

- anxiety
- confusion
- emotional instability
- headaches
- inability to cope
- nervousness
- irritability
- faintness and dizziness

- antisocial behavior
- depression
- exhaustion
- impatience
- intense hunger
- phobias
- sugar craving
- mental confusion

Causes

Stress can cause hypoglycemia. There are many, many stressors in our modern day lives. Some are physical; injuries, environmental noise and pollution, temperature extremes, etc. Others are social; death, divorce, or loss of a job. There are happy stressful occurrences such as birth of a baby, a marriage, or a promotion in a job. These, however, still put a strain on your psychological and physiological well-being. Another area of stress can be psychological. Fear, worry, hate and other negative emotions put a burden on the body. These all take their toll on our nervous systems. Financial worry is a very real and common source of frustration and tension in this day and age. Disharmony among families or associates provokes much stress, which sets the stage for illness — both mental and physical. Often we cannot control what happens or when. Therefore, it is extremely important that we fortify our bodies nutritionally so that when life-shaking conditions threaten us we will not "fall apart."

Stress affects different people in various ways. Studies show it is a primary cause of disease. Free radicals are fragmentary molecules which are released when a person is under severe stress. They create lesions in the nervous system and are potent and dangerous irritants to the entire body. The adrenal glands are the "stress glands" of the body. They must react to any demand placed on them. They become burdened when a person is constantly subjected to relentless stress, and eventually become exhausted. Symptoms of adrenal exhaustion include chronic fatigue, irritability, depression, low stress tolerance, the feeling of being unable to cope, nervous exhaustion, insomnia, and difficulty in relaxing, as well as hypoglycemia.

Poor dietary choices are the main cause of hypoglycemia. A diet high in refined foods and excessive sugar exhausts the adrenals. White sugar is not a food; it is a chemical which wears out the glandular system. The adrenals and pancreas are over-stressed when refined starches, sugars, and a high meat diet are consumed. Sugar is an addictive substance, and the low blood sugar state, which you get from eating it, makes the cravings more intense. The food industry has discovered that increasing the sugar content in products increases the amount a person will eat, which will increase sales. Some doctors feel that if hypoglycemia goes untreated for a long period of time it can develop into diabetes.

The adrenals can become exhausted from the combination of stress, worry, and the toxic accumulation of undigested starches, sugars, proteins and dairy products. This depletes the cortin hormone and the ability to digest food properly. Alcohol, drugs, cigarettes, caffeine, chemical food additives, deadline pressures, inadequate sleep, etc. can also contribute to this problem. Glandular dysfunction and mineral deficiencies are other causes. Heavy metal poisoning can produce hypoglycemia. Stress will uncover weaknesses and imbalances in various organs of the body. It will affect these weak organs in various ways. A sick colon, for instance, may manifest itself under stress, with diarrhea. Tension will place an undue burden on any weak area of the body and make it more vulnerable to disease.

Hans Selye, an early pioneer in stress research, discovered a relationship between stress and physiological response. This response is a chain reaction which starts in the hypothalamus area of the brain. This stimulates the pituitary gland to generate hormones, which regulate the endocrine system. The adrenals are part of this endocrine network. The adrenals release the hormone "adrenaline" and a group of hormones known as corticosteroids. One of these corticosteroids is called "hydrocortisone" or "cortisol." Elevated levels of cortisol suppress the immune system by debilitating the beneficial T-cells and reducing the virus-killer interferon. Health author Dr. Michael A. Weiner, explains: "A wide range of diseases are associated with elevated cortisol levels, including depression, cancer, hypertension, ulcers, heart attack, diabetes, cancer, hypertension, ulcers, heart attack, diabetes, infections, alcoholism, obesity, arthritis, stroke, psychoses of the aging, skin diseases, Parkinson's disease, multiple sclerosis, myasthenia gravis and even perhaps Alzheimer's disease. Elevated levels of cortisol are even reported to be a useful predictor of suicide."

NATURAL TREATMENT

The following should be eliminated from the diet: nicotine, caffeine, theobromine, theophylline, purines found in animal products, coffee, meat, and tea. Chocolate contains toxic alkaloids that damage the pancreas. They interfere with glandular function and create addictions.

Carbonated drinks interfere with digestion. Stomach problems are common with hypoglycemia. Avoid heavy fat diets and fried foods. They cause a lowering of blood sugar and a reduction of sugar in the urine. Avoid an excess of dairy products; they are constipating and are high in lactose (milk sugar).

Read labels when purchasing food. The following are forms of sugars: dextrose, dextrin, maltose, lactose, sucrose, fructose, modified food starch, cornstarch, corn syrup, corn sweetener, natural sweetener, honey (use in small amounts), and molasses (use in small amounts). The following are forms of alcohol and react in the body with refined carbohydrates: sorbitol, mannitol, hexitol and glycol.

DIETARY GUIDELINES

Avoid too much table salt. It creates adrenal exhaustion and causes a loss of potassium, which leads to a drop in blood sugar. Eat natural foods and eliminate the ones that caused the problems in the first place. White flour and white sugar products, refined and processed foods, fast foods cooked in rancid oils, heavy meat diets, ice cream, pastries, cookies, candy, processed cereals, soft drinks, and caffeine products should be eliminated.

Eat small meals throughout the day. Learn stress reduction. Increase the intake of whole grains (millet, buckwheat, rye, wheat, and barley). Use beans, raw seeds, nuts, vegetables and fruit. Sprouts are rich in nutrients. Grains digest slowly and release sugar into the bloodstream gradually for as long as 6 to 8 hours after the meal. The complex carbohydrates in grains help to keep blood sugar levels constant for a long period of time.

NUTRITIONAL SUPPLEMENTS

Licorice root acts in the body like the cortin hormone and protects the adrenal glands, helping them to cope with stress. It stabilizes blood sugar levels and provides a feeling of well-being.

Alfalfa provides vegetable protein to nourish the adrenal glands.

Cedar Berries heal and nourish the pancreas.

Goldenseal helps regulate blood sugar levels.

Vitamin A assists in maintaining normal glandular function.

B-complex vitamins are necessary to control the mood swings associated with hypoglycemia. They build the adrenals and calm the nerves.

Vitamin C with bioflavonoids helps to prevent low blood-sugar attacks.

Vitamin E protects B-vitamins from rapid oxidation and reduces cholesterol. It is necessary for rebuilding the adrenal and pituitary glands.

Calcium and magnesium help prevent adrenal instability. They work with vitamins A, C and E, zinc and inositol for proper absorption.

Chromium is essential for proper metabolism of sugar.

Iodine regulates hormones to control metabolism.

Manganese assists in pancreatic development and in maintenance of healthy nerves.

Acidophilus is beneficial for improving digestion.

Blue-green algae and Chlorophyll are cleansing and healing.

Germanium and Co Q-10 help provide oxygen to the blood vessels and cells.

Essential fatty acids serve as precursors to hormone-like substances that help regulate every body function.

FACTS AT A GLANCE

• Stress and poor eating habits can contribute to hypoglycemia.
• Avoiding junk foods and stimulants will help regulate blood flow.
• Getting proper rest allows the body and its organs to rest.
• Take supplements that strengthen the adrenal glands.

Hypothyroidism

Hypothyroidism exists when the thyroid gland is underactive and does not produce enough of the hormone thyroxine. It can be hereditary or it may result from an iodine deficiency. The thyroid needs iodine to function normally. Without the proper amount of iodine the gland cannot manufacture the normal quantity of thyroxine.

The thyroid is a small butterfly-shaped gland located in the neck and weighs less than an ounce. The thyroid controls the metabolism that transforms food into energy. It regulates the rate at which the body utilizes oxygen and controls the rate which various organs function. Every organ, tissue and cell is affected by the hormone secretions of the thyroid gland. Dr. Broda O. Barnes, author of *Hypothyroidism: The Unsuspected Illness*, states: "Of all the sly, subtle problems that can affect physical or mental health, none is more common than thyroid gland disturbances."

Symptoms

It is a well-known fact that hypothyroidism can have a mental and emotional effect on the body. The following are only a few of the many problems associated with hypothyroidism:

- anemia
- concentration difficulties
- depression
- headaches
- high blood pressure
- insomnia
- menstrual problems
- recurrent infections
- weight gain
- cold feeling (poor circulation)
- constipation
- hair loss
- heart problems
- infections
- low back pain
- muscle cramps and weakness
- skin problems

The following is a self-test developed by Dr. Barnes. Take a thermometer and shake it down and put it on your bedstand. Immediately upon awakening in the morning, place the thermometer snugly in the armpit for ten minutes. A reading below the normal range of 97.8 to 98.2 strongly suggests low thyroid function. If the reading is above the normal range, one may suspect some infection or an overactive thyroid gland.

Causes

Thyroid function may become imbalanced when the body is encumbered with toxins, mucus waste, and/or inadequate nutrition, particularly a lack of iodine. The need for iodine seems to increase when infection invades the body. Using natural herbs like kelp or dulse will regulate the gland, whether it is underactive or overactive.

Cooked food kills enzymes and causes the endocrine glands to become overworked, leading to body toxicity and a disturbance in glandular function. Cooked food overstimulates the thyroid gland and causes the body to retain excess weight. When the glands do not receive the nutrients necessary to satisfy the body's needs, they overstimulate the digestive organs and demand more food because the body is not satisfied. This produces an oversecretion of hormones and an unhealthy appetite, which finally results in exhaustion of the hormone-producing glands. The enzymes from live food help the body to maintain proper metabolism. Besides an inadequate or junk food diet, hypothyroidism can also be caused by chemicals found in the food and water supply, poor absorption of nutrients in the body and systemic candidiasis (yeast infection throughout the body).

NATURAL TREATMENT AND DIETARY GUIDELINES

Eat live foods such as sprouts, salads, raw fruits and vegetables. Thermos-cooked grains and rice help retain nutrients. Raw, unsalted seeds and nuts (sesame seeds, pumpkin seeds, sunflower seeds, almonds, pecans,and cashews) are nutritious. Raw vegetable juices (carrot, celery, parsley and comfrey) and green drinks containing chlorophyll help nourish the thyroid gland and entire system.

Avoid all junk foods. They overstimulate the glands and cause exhaustion and weakness. Sugar and white flour products are detrimental. Fried foods are hard to digest and cause the formation of free radicals, which destroy the cells. Avoid all drugs, especially oral contraceptives, antibiotics, sulfa drugs and tranquilizers. They will put a burden on the glands and cause dysfunction.

NUTRITIONAL SUPPLEMENTS

Irish Moss contains all the essential minerals for a healthy thyroid, such as potassium, magnesium, iodine, chlorine and sodium, plus many more. It has the ability of changing the chemistry of the body from disease to health. It is useful to all the functions of the body. Irish moss contains calcium sulfate which helps clean out the accumulation of abnormal growths in the tissues. It causes the infiltrated parts to discharge their contents so they do not lay dormant and slowly decay. The properties of Irish moss are: demulcent (soothing mucilage substance used internally to protect damaged or inflamed tissues), emollient (softening, soothing and protective) and a nutritive tonic (helps provide a general effect on the entire body).

Kelp supplies all the essential minerals to the body in an easily assimilated form. It is rich in iodine which is so necessary for healthy thyroid function, as well as strengthening to the nervous system and brain. It is said to be essential during pregnancy. Kelp is rich in natural sodium, which helps calcium to be absorbed properly in the system. It is an excellent promoter of glandular health, which includes the thyroid, pituitary and adrenals. Kelp contains every vital mineral needed for sustaining bodily health.

Black Walnut helps the body to withstand stressful conditions. It is rich in potassium and iodine, which contain very healing and antiseptic properties. Black walnut oxygenates the blood, kills parasites and helps balance blood sugar levels.

Watercress is very useful as a tonic to help regulate the metabolism and the flow of bile. Watercress is rich in vitamins A, C, and D, and is one of the best plant sources of vitamin E. It is high in minerals to feed the glands, especially iodine, calcium, manganese, copper and sulphur.

Cat's Claw [also known as uña de gato] helps eliminate yeast infections and parasites in the body. It has antioxidant and anti-inflammatory properties, among many other benefits.

FACTS AT A GLANCE

• Hypothyroidism can have both a mental and emotional effect on the body.
• Eat "live" foods.
• Avoid junk foods.
• Herbs that nourish the thyroid include kelp and Irish moss.

Obesity

When we come to understand how harmful being overweight is on our bodies, and how it can predispose us to diabetes, heart disease, strokes and many other illnesses, then we will realize how vital it is to control our eating habits. The American way of eating has given us an unhealthy appetite for refined, harmful foods. We cannot even call them food, for they don't even satisfy our body's need for nutrition. If they did, our appetites wouldn't be out of control.

Symptoms

"Mirror, mirror, on the wall . . ."

Causes

When we start eating nutritional food, this alone will control our appetites. Our bodies will tell us, "Hey, you have given me the vitamins and minerals I need, so I won't need to beg for more." The body has a natural appestat mechanism in the brain telling when we have eaten enough, but because it has been distorted, we become obese. We have not listened to our body. We have essentially destroyed the ability of our own bodies to warn us when to stop eating. And now, because our appestat is not working properly, it is time for us to get control of ourselves and work toward losing weight.

Lack of exercise has a negative effect on appestat mechanisms. You know how our beef and poultry are fattened up? They are kept in close quarters and given hormones to make them become fatter in a shorter period, so more money can be made. Autointoxication is another reason for obesity. Our bodies are not able to eliminate each day all the waste material, and it will build up and cause weight gain. The following are specific areas in which obesity may be caused:

Stress: It is difficult for some individuals to lose weight when they are under stress, because they want to eat a lot to comfort themselves. It is best to try to cope with stress in other ways, such as getting involved in recreation and hobbies.

Depression: When problems and difficulties arise, some people plunge into an abyss of despair. This is especially true when the situation is already depressing and the self-image is at a low ebb. This also encourages extra eating and sitting at home, brooding. The best remedy is to get out and associate with upbeat people.

Nutritional Deficiencies: Your entire well-being is dependent upon excellent nutrition. Your glands especially need to be nourished so they can serve you. Inadequate nutrition will cause an imbalance in your body and you will find it harder to lose weight.

Parasites: There is increasing evidence that parasites and other organisms may play a part in overeating. The body is constantly being robbed of essential nutrients when it harbors these unwelcome visitors. As a result, the body craves more food to compensate for the nutrient loss and overeating becomes a vicious cycle. There are herbs (such as black walnut) which will kill parasites and remove them from the body.

Candida yeast infection: Yeast can produce toxins that inhibit the conversions of sugars and fats to energy. (For more information, please see section on *Candida albicans*).

Lack of enzymes: Eating a diet high in cooked foods, versus eating one consisting mainly of raw foods, can contribute to weight gain. In the book *Enzyme Nutrition,* Dr. Edward Howell explains:

> Raw calories are relatively non-stimulating to glands, and tend to stabilize weight. Cooked calories excite glands and tend to be fattening. I am not here referring to something like a dish of cooked spinach, which has few calories in the first place. But a slice of bread or a boiled potato stimulates glands and will put on the ounces which add into many pounds. Let us learn something from animals. Technical men in the business of extracting the maximum profit from farm animals found it was not economical to feed hogs raw potatoes. The hogs would not get fat enough. Cooking the potatoes, however, produced the fat hogs that brought the farmer the kind of money required to make a profit. This in spite of the extra expense of labor and energy involved in cooking!

> Avocados are blessed with a lot of nice calories. Ever hear of anyone getting fat on them? Or on bananas, which also have plenty of raw calories? It would be an exceptional person who could eat enough bananas to get fat. All of these high-calorie raw foods might fill out a thin individual to a slight degree, but they know just where to put the ounces and when to stop. They will not drape the weight about in ugly disarray over the exterior, or clog up delicate heart arteries...To judge a banana, an avocado, an apple, or an orange by its calories is

just as misleading and false as evaluating the moral stature of a pretty woman by her exterior embellishments. There is a difference between raw and cooked calories . . .

NATURAL TREATMENT

Exercise is a key factor. Exercise promotes circulation, which is an important factor in how we feel. It improves the quality of our blood. Glandular function is improved with exercise, which releases hormones necessary for health and appetite control. We need to understand the process of digestion, which prepares nutrients for assimilation through the wall of the small intestines into the bloodstream. When we learn more about our bodies, we will become convinced that going on a diet is not the answer. The answer is to change our habits, whether it is food, exercise, or how we feel about ourselves.

Through the years, many women have tried chemical drugs in their quest for weight loss. They work by artificially speeding up the metabolism and/or manipulating neurotransmitters in the brain. Currently, the two most popular weight-loss drugs are Pondimin® (fenfluramine) and Fastin® (phentermine). They are usually prescribed together. Even doctors admit "they do not seem to cause a permanent lowering of the set point. Some patients who stop them will show weight gain. Those who exercise and diet carefully may be able to maintain some or all of their weight loss if they stop the medication." Minor side-effects may include: dry mouth, diarrhea, blurred vision, sleepiness, insomnia, constipation, palpitations, depression, vivid dreams, dizziness, and elevated blood pressure. Major side effects include short-term memory loss, shortness of breath, and agitation. We prefer the natural approach because it works *with* the body, instead of tricking it. This way, you do not have to worry about side effects, some of which are very harmful.

Blood purification, lower bowel cleansing and lymphatic cleansing will help clean the cells. It may take a year, but when the bloodstream and tissues are purified, the glands will function properly and you will see the weight come off naturally. Obesity is a chronic condition, and it may take patience and time. However, you will feel so much better, and your whole body will feel clean and healthy. A healthy body produces a healthy mind.

DIETARY GUIDELINES

A major portion of the diet should consist of fruits and vegetables. Fruits are the cleansers of the body and vegetables are the builders. Lightly steamed vegetables will provide minerals. High-fiber foods are essential. Proper chewing will cut the appetite. Carrot, celery, beet and apple juice are needed to feed the glands. Lemon juice in a glass of water first thing in the morning will cleanse the liver, which helps filter toxins. Nutritious foods to consider include green leafy vegetables, carrots, broccoli, celery, tomatoes, apples, cantaloupe, berries, melons, plums, almonds, sesame seeds, asparagus, and cabbage. Whole grains, steamed in a thermos overnight, retain enzymes which help the body with digestion and assimilation.

It is wise to establish a regular eating routine. Try to eat at the same time every day. You do not need three giant meals per day. Remember the adage, "Breakfast like a king (or queen!), lunch like a prince (or princess), and supper like a pauper." This is best for your digestion, metabolism and calorie-utilization. Plan out a menu and when you shop become a "label-reader." Look for hidden sugars in the foods, such as corn syrup, dextrose, etc. Next, study and learn as much as you can about nutrition. Learn about vitamins, minerals, etc., and what they do for your body. Fourth, substitute some foods in your diet. Learn to replace salt with kelp or vegetable seasoning. We get too much table salt in our modern foods, anyway. Excessive salt can lead to water-retention, high blood pressure, potassium imbalance and many other problems. Pepper is irritating to the stomach. Use onions, garlic, and bell peppers to flavor and season foods. Also, there are many herbs to select from, such as rosemary, thyme, basil, etc. Fifth, eat moderately, but do not starve yourself. Watching calories and measuring them is self-defeating. Forget about calories. Concentrate instead on the delicious array of nutritious foods from which you have to choose.

Excessive sugar and starch create an abnormal appetite. This dangerous combination affects the body chemically like alcohol. The more it is used, the more the craving increases. Sugar hastens decay or fermentation and acid is rapidly produced. Use honey sparingly for sweetening. A little goes a long way. Ten to twelve glasses of pure water daily (four glasses in succession) can "jolt" the body's metabolism into a higher gear. Any other liquids (juice, herbal teas, etc.) do not count. It has to be plain old water. This will also expedite the body's release of the toxins which keep fat in the cells.

NUTRITIONAL SUPPLEMENTS

Burdock helps the pituitary gland adjust hormone balance in the body. A malfunctioning pituitary gland can contribute to being overweight.

Echinacea cleanses the body of toxins without any side effects. When the body is free of poisons, it is better able to balance itself in other areas, among them weight regulation.

Sarsaparilla is often used in herbal formulas to balance the glands. It has stimulating properties which have been helpful in increasing metabolic rate.

Black Walnut promotes oxygen in the blood, which will kill parasites. It will help balance sugar levels and is able to assist the body in burning up excessive toxins and fatty materials.

Goldenseal stimulates a sluggish glandular system and balances the hormones. It helps regulate liver functions. The natural antibiotic properties will stop infection and kill poisons in the body. If a person has low blood sugar, substitute myrrh instead.

Chickweed is an effective appetite suppressant, blood purifier, and fat-burner. It also has diuretic properties.

Garcinia cambogia is a fruit from a plant native to India that accelerates the rate at which fat within the cells is burned.

Chinese ephedra creates a condition known as thermogenesis, where the body temperature and metabolism is increased. This promotes the body's ability to burn fat.

Kelp is an excellent promoter of healthy glands and regulates the metabolism which helps digest food. It speeds up the burning of excess calories. It is very nourishing to the entire body, especially the adrenal, pituitary and thyroid glands. Kelp contains all of the minerals considered vital to health. It helps the nervous system. It is beneficial to the brain and stimulates it to function normally. Kelp contains nearly 30 minerals.

Digestive enzymes will help the body process and assimilate food, ensuring that it gets maximum nutrition and utilizes fats and sugars properly.

FACTS AT A GLANCE

• Diets generally do not work well for permanent, healthy weight-loss.
• Exercise is important for keeping weight off.
• Changing diets to include nutritional foods is essential.

Cellulite

Cellulite is the excess fat that looks like lumps, bumps or dimple deposits on the hips, thighs and buttocks. Cellulite is most often found in women.

CAUSES

Cellulite is caused by lack of exercise, too many starches and sweets, and the wrong kinds of fats. This is most often found in women who produce extra estrogen. When the liver cannot excrete the estrogen properly, it encourages fat accumulation in the wrong places.

Fatty buildup in the tissues results from an underactive bowel created by poor nutrition and elimination, whether or not you have one or two bowel movements a day.

Poor lymphatic drainage can be a problem and exercise can help. Fat can be trapped between the cells where they are held by hardened connective tissues which collect pockets of water, toxins, and fat that gives the skin the puckered appearance.

NATURAL TREATMENT

A lasting approach to eliminating cellulite consists of changing one's lifestyle, keeping the colon functioning properly and eating a diet high in raw fruits and vegetables. Cellulite is ugly, unwanted fat and is very hard to eliminate, but with desire and determination it can be done. Skin brushing will also speed up the elimination of cellulite. Skin brushing is a well-known and proven method for encouraging better lymphatic circulation. Brushing with a long-handled, natural bristle or a loofah "sponge" creates surface friction which promotes circulation and brings nourishment to the skin.

DIETARY GUIDELINES

Cleaning the colon and adopting a high-fiber natural diet are essential. Eat plenty of fresh fruits and vegetables. Use whole grains, such as brown rice, millet, whole oats, kamut, spelt, amaranth and buckwheat.

NUTRITIONAL SUPPLEMENTS

B-complex Vitamins help to eradicate cellulite, especially B3 and niacin, which improve circulation and help lower blood fats.
Vitamin E and Lecithin help emulsify cholesterol.
Vitamin C, Potassium and B6 will speed up the elimination of cellulite.
Acidophilus helps utilize nutrients.
Blue-green Algae and Chlorophyll help clean blood and nourish the skin.
Flaxseed Oil and Salmon Oil help burn excessive fat in cells.
Co Q-10 and Germanium help supply oxygen to the cells.

FACTS AT A GLANCE

- Regular exercise will prevent snacking by balancing the "appestat."
- Good nutrition plays an integral role in weight loss. Avoid junk foods.
- Eating at a regular time each day can help put the body in balance.
- Proper supplementation can help naturally increase the body's metabolism.

engers, waiting for the opportunity to invade the filth in the system. Viruses cannot produce on their own. They need a host to survive. A germ is a bacterium. It is easily seen with an ordinary microscope. It multiplies and spreads by itself, given the proper conditions. The body can recognize a germ and alerts the macrophages or "germ eaters" of the immune system that the foreign organism has invaded the body's territory. The macrophage then "eats" the germ and gets rid of it. When the macrophage (which is a white blood cell) eats enough germs, it has done its duty and then dies. When there is an accumulation of these dead macrophages, it creates the substance known as pus.

Viruses are a different story. They are very sneaky. The word *virus* comes from the Latin word for "slimy liquid" or "poison." Viruses are very selective about choosing their hosts. Some viruses, like those which cause the flu or rabies, can infect either humans or animals, but most favor certain cells or species. "If it's AIDS, it commonly goes to the T-cells," states Dr. Bernard Fields, chairman of the department of microbiology and molecular genetics at Harvard University. "If it's polio, it goes to certain subsets of nerve cells in the spinal cord. If it's hepatitis, it goes to the liver."

Viruses are very tiny in comparison to germs. The difference has been likened in size to a pin head beside a basketball. Viruses are ten to one hundred times as tiny as the average bacterium. They can only be detected by an electron microscope.

How do viruses know which cells they can invade? The answer lies in the protein shell that encases the virus. The protein shell has markers on its exterior which mesh exactly with the receptors found on the surface of certain cells. The virus attaches itself to specific areas on the cell's exterior, is then covered by part of the cell's membrane and taken inside, like a guest. Some viruses use other means to enter the host cells. Once the virus is inside the cell, it sheds its protein coat and integrates its DNA with the host cell's genetic code. The cell does nothing to extricate the virus, believing it is part of itself. Once the genetic reprogramming is set in motion, the cell's genetic apparatus reproduces viruses over and over again. This reaction ultimately leads to the host cell's demise, because eventually the viruses multiply to the extent that it bursts the cell and destroys it. The virus invades more cells and promotes additional destruction of the body's defenses. The key to avoiding the harmful microbes is embracing positive health habits.

Cancer

Much of the following information is taken from *The Complete Home Health Advisor*, by Rita Elkins.

Cancer has become a byword of the 20th century. Living in fear of contracting cancer is not uncommon due to the vast number of carcinogenic substances to which modern life exposes us, not to mention harmful lifestyles which many of us choose to live. Cancer is a term which refers to over 100 different diseases in which there is an unrestrained growth of cells, either within an organ or in the tissues. Benign tumors, unlike malignant ones, do not spread and infiltrate the surrounding tissue. Cells from a malignant tumor may spread (metastasize) through the blood vessels and lymph system to other parts of the body, in which new tumors will continue to grow.

Areas in the body where malignant tumors most commonly develop are lungs, breasts, stomach, colon, skin, pancreas, liver, prostate, uterus, ovaries, bone marrow, the lymphatic system, bones or muscles. Carcinomas are cancers of the skin, mucuous membranes, glands and organs. Leukemias are blood cancers. Sarcomas refer to cancers of the muscles, connective tissues, and the bones. Lymphomas attack the lymphatic system. (For additional information on estrogen-dependent cancers, please refer to the chapter on Estrogen). Cancer ranks as the second most common cause of death in the United States, with heart disease as the first.

Symptoms

- a sore that does not heal
- nagging cough or chronic hoarseness
- coughing up bloody sputum
- a change in a wart or mole
- difficulty swallowing

- chronic indigestion
- a thickening or lump in the breast or any other part of the body
- bleeding or discharge, bleeding between menstrual periods
- obvious changes in bowel or bladder habits
- blood in the stool
- a persistent low-grade fever
- headaches accompanied by visual disturbances
- unusual fatigue
- excessive bruising
- repeated nosebleeds
- loss of appetite and weight loss
- persistent abdominal pain
- blood in the urine with no pain during urination
- continuous unexplained back pain

CAUSES

Thirty years ago, one in twenty contracted cancer. Today it is one in three. The type of food we eat can gradually create a toxic condition in the body that invites cancer cells to grow. Cancer has a long incubation period which can last many years. Building up the immune system is necessary so the body can heal itself.

Some studies have suggested that if cells are deprived of oxygen, they may become prone to malignant growth. Consequently, because the blood provides all cells with oxygen, the condition of the bloodstream is important in the treatment and prevention of cancer. Vitamins, minerals and herbs which help in facilitating circulation and detoxification of the blood are very important.

The National Academy of Sciences has recently validated what several nutritionally oriented practitioners have said for years: that there is a link between diet and cancer. A high-fiber, low-fat diet is now accepted as a valid deterrent to some types of cancer. In addition, animal fats, high-sugar diets, caffeine and alcohol may increase your risk of several forms of cancer.

The main cause of cancer is the presence of poisons or toxins in the bloodstream. The cancer growth acts as a dumping encasement for the poisons. The cancer indicates that the blood is overloaded and is unable to eliminate in the normal way because of constipation and autointoxication.

Cancerous growths require sugar to grow. Rancid oils and fats are dangerous, for they decrease oxygenation, inhibiting the function of every cell. Rancid oils and heavy protein diets cause the blood to become heavy and thickened and limits its transport ability. When the blood is too thick, the elimination organs (the liver, kidneys, bowels and skin) have a difficult time doing their job. Researchers in Sweden estimate that 30 to 40 percent of cancer in males and 60 percent of cancer in females is caused by dietary deficiencies.

NATURAL TREATMENT

Good nutrition and detoxification will speed the elimination of toxins which destroy the organs that build and clean the blood. Dietary indoles reduce the risk of breast, cervical and colon cancers. Fresh juice fasting and wheatgrass juice inhibit cancer cells.

DIETARY GUIDELINES

Avoid the following foods: saturated fats, salt, sugar, alcohol, coffee, caffeine, and animal proteins. Avoid meat, which is dead matter, cut out fats and eliminate salt-cured, salt-pickled and smoked foods such as sausage, bacon, ham, smoked fish, bologna and hot dogs. Restrict dairy foods.

A macrobiotic diet has been used by some cancer patients, who claim good results. It involves eating brown rice and certain vegetables. Eat a low-fat diet high in fiber and complex carbohydrates. Sprouted grains are rich in vitamins and minerals. Cruciferous vegetables such as cabbage, broccoli, brussels sprouts and cauliflower protect against cancer and contain plant nutrients known as indoles, which prevent the formation of cancer in the intestines. Foods rich in potassium, such as beans, sprouts, whole grains, almonds, sunflower seeds, sesame seeds, lentils, parsley, blueberries, coconut, endive, leaf lettuce, oats, potatoes with skins, carrots and peaches are also suggested in designing an anticancer diet.

Eat a diet high in raw fruits and vegetables, raw seeds and nuts, and drink plenty of freshly squeezed juices such as carrot, apple, spinach and kale. Keep the bowels active by eating soaked figs, prunes or raisins.

Fluoride in water and toothpaste is linked to bone cancer. Breathing unhealthy air causes cancer.

NUTRITIONAL SUPPLEMENTS

Beta Carotene is a strong antioxidant that can help destroy free radicals in the body.

Garlic in capsule form can enhance immune function. It also acts as a natural antibiotic.

Germanium and Coenzyme Q-10 help to enhance cellular oxygenation and stimulates the immune system. They can also help to relieve pain.

Selenium helps to properly digest proteins.

Vitamins A and E are important for proper immune function. Both of these vitamins also participate in damaged tissue repair and regeneration.

Vitamin B complex helps maintain normal cell division and cell function.

Vitamin C with bioflavonoids is considered an anticarcinogen and can help to detoxify the system.

Vitamin D helps the body utilize calcium, vitamin A and essential minerals.

Calcium and Magnesium supplement with silicon and zinc is important for the proper function of nerves and muscles.

Chlorophyll obtained through wheatgrass juice is thought to help boost red blood cell development, which serves to oxygenate tissue.

Cat's Claw (uña de gato) helps stimulate the body's production of macrophages (white blood cells) and helps activate them to eliminate foreign invaders such as bacteria, viruses and other toxins.

Essential Fatty Acids (such as evening primrose oil, borage oil, flaxseed oil, etc.) have demonstrated through studies to inhibit the growth of cancer, especially breast cancer.

Pau d'Arco (taheebo) tea helps to protect the liver and is especially recommended if taking chemotherapy or radiation treatments.

Burdock helps to cleanse the blood and remove toxins, which can result from the cancer and from radiation and chemotherapy.

Dandelion helps to clear the blood of toxins and is an excellent liver stimulant. The liver detoxifies the system of drugs, radiation effects, etc., and must be kept as healthy as possible.

Echinacea boosts the body's immune defenses.

Suma works to help strengthen the entire system.

Red Clover has been used as an anticancer agent since the 1930s.

FACTS AT A GLANCE

- Cancer is the second most common cause of death in the United States.
- Cancer usually has a long incubation period.
- Detoxification of the blood is imperative to preventing cancer.
- Oxygenation of the cells is vital (cancer cells cannot thrive in the presence of oxygen).

Allergies

Allergies come in many forms and can affect any part of the body, even the brain. More people are bothered by allergies today than any other time in history. Allergies became especially recognized at the turn of the century when we became a technologically advanced nation, with hidden additives in our food, antibiotics and hormones added to our beef and poultry. Fruits and vegetables are sprayed so that they can be shipped all over the nation and still appeal to the eye. We are burdened with an ever-increasing rate of toxic wastes in the air and water. Over 3,000 additives and preservatives are added to our food. Take time to look at the boxed food labels at the supermarket.

Allergies afflict the majority of people at different times. Most of these individuals are unaware that what they are suffering is allergy-related. Recently, reactions beyond red eyes and sniffles have been linked to allergies. Some include digestion problems, hyperactivity, attention problems, mental illness, arthritis and many more.

SYMPTOMS

- acne, blisters, blotches, circles under the eyes, eczema, flushing, hives, itching, and psoriasis
- high blood pressure, hypertension, low blood pressure, irregular heartbeat, and rapid pulse (very common when allergic to ingested food)
- headaches (variety), confusion, mental dullness, depression, crying, anger, anxiety, irritability, learning and memory difficulties, lack of concentration, restlessness, fatigue, and insomnia
- arthritis, muscle cramps, spasm and joint pain, extreme fatigue, sluggishness, neck, back or shoulder aches, and lack of coordination
- asthma, cough, frequent colds, hay fever, mouth breathing, nose bleeds, post nasal drip, wheezing, shortness of breath, tightness in chest, and rattling sounds in chest
- constipation, colitis, canker sores, peptic ulcers, diarrhea, stomach cramps, nausea, heartburn, food cravings, indigestion, hemorrhoids, bloating, and vomiting
- bed-wetting, overweight, hypoglycemia, and glandular diseases

CAUSES

Allergies are caused primarily by poor diet, which causes digestion and assimilation problems; they are also caused by toxins being absorbed into the blood and lymphatic system, causing excess mucus, as well as undigested protein, viruses, germs, parasites and worms. We have worn out our digestive system, immune system and glands.

Leaky gut syndrome is a common problem connected with allergies. Large spaces develop between the cells of the gut wall and allow viruses, bacteria, toxins and food to enter and get into the blood.

Undigested proteins act as irritants in the body. The cells treat them as foreign invaders, thus inviting an "allergic attack." An efficient digestive system is necessary to prevent accumulation of these substances in the bloodstream.

The colon, which is the "intestinal" part of the system, plays a vital function in preventing allergies. Its role is to eliminate waste material. However, due to faulty eating habits, eating junk food, wrong combining of food, too much meat, white flour and sugar products and an unbalanced diet, the colon becomes congested or "constipated." It will then harbor all manner of toxins, which will poison and irritate different parts of the body when released into the bloodstream. This state of autointoxication lowers the immune capability of the body and sets the stage or condition for allergies to occur.

Lack of digestive enzymes is another cause of allergies. Enzymes are essential to prevent immune system disorders. A Russian scientist named Kouchadoff discovered that after cooked food is eaten, white blood cells increase in the intestines. The white cells, which are part of the immune system, always increase in number when there is a need to eliminate hostile invaders. Their extra concentration indicates the start of an inflammation or disease. In other words, cooked food places an added strain on the glands and immune system. But when raw food is eaten the white cells do not increase.

NATURAL TREATMENT

A change of diet is necessary. An allergy usually builds up gradually, and may be caused by the same foods you eat every day. Change to a more healthy diet. Drinking 8 to 10 glasses of distilled water every day will help to eliminate toxins. Fasting is a beneficial way to restore health to the digestive system. Fresh vegetable and fruit juices, with their live enzymes, will nourish and heal the digestive tract.

Eliminate red meat, sugar, white flour products, dairy products, (except live culture or plain yogurt), and all refined food.

Parasites can be a problem when allergies are present. Black walnut, wormwood, and pumpkin seeds, are some of the herbs that will eliminate worms and parasites.

An herbal formula that will clean and heal the lining of the digestive tract should contain some the following herbs: gentian, goldenseal, myrrh, Irish moss, fenugreek, comfrey, prickly ash, blue vervain, St. John's wort and mandrake.

Herbal formulas to clean the colon and blood are very beneficial. A liver cleanse is beneficial, when the liver is congested with fats and toxins, it cannot protect the body from allergies.

DIETARY GUIDELINES

Eat fruit alone. When eaten first thing in the morning it will help the body cleanse from fasting all night. A good liver cleanse in the morning is a cup of warm water with the juice of a lemon or lime, grated ginger, fenugreek powder, licorice powder and a teaspoon of pure olive oil. Mix in blender an drink first thing in the morning.

Food combining will take stress off the digestive tract, and give it a chance to heal. Whole grains can be eaten with all steamed vegetables and salads. Eat some fish and chicken (organic) with vegetables (except potatoes). A baked potato can be eaten with vegetables.

Brown basmati rice and millet can be cooked together and used in your favorite dishes or eaten as a cereal. They are easy to digest and healing to the digestive tract.

Drink nut and seed milk. Almonds soaked for twenty-four hours and blended can be used instead of milk.

Eat sprouts. They benefit the digestive tract and contain enzymes, vitamins and minerals. Alfalfa, fenugreek and radish make an excellent blend.

Green drinks will help cleanse the blood and cells. Wheatgrass juice is a very powerful cleanser. Barley grass juice is also beneficial. An excellent juice combination for cleaning is made from carrot, celery, and a handful of endive, garlic and fresh ginger.

NUTRITIONAL SUPPLEMENTS

Acidophilus helps to balance the good and bad bacteria in the intestines. It also helps in digestion and assimilation.

Chlorophyll and Blue-green Algae help restore health to the immune system. They are cleansing and contain a rich amount of nutrients. They also break down poisonous carbon dioxide.

Vitamin A is necessary to digest and utilize protein, and for healthy mucous membranes to help wash away allergy-causing toxins.

Vitamin E protects the fat in the cell membranes from rancidity. (Rancid fat causes holes in the cell membranes through which allergens enter and cause reactions.)

Bee Pollen can help build immunity by nourishing membranes that act as a barrier against inhaled pollen and other toxins. It is rich in protein.

B-complex Vitamins are essential for the general health of the adrenal glands and can be effective in guarding against allergic reactions. B6 has antihistamine effects.

Vitamin C with bioflavonoids work together to act as a natural antihistamine to prevent foreign substances from entering the body. 5,000 milligrams or more daily, along with B-vitamins, help in blocking allergic reactions as well as rebuilding healthy membranes.

Calcium and Magnesium must be balanced. A combination providing half as much magnesium as calcium is ideal. They have an anti-allergic effect and may be helpful to repair damage done to the cell membranes which occur as a result of allergic reactions. This duo cleans the blood, regulates heartbeat, helps alleviate insomnia and protects the nervous system.

Essential Fatty Acids help the body produce prostaglandins which help reduce inflammation. They are found in oils such as flaxseed, borage, black currant, evening primrose and salmon.

Minerals are essential for all functions of the body and work with vitamins to build and strengthen all systems. Zinc selenium, boron, and silicon are especially important for women. They help protect the bones.

FACTS AT A GLANCE

- Allergies are very widespread and can go undetected.
- There are many diseases where the underlying cause are allergies, because of the lack of enzymes.
- A cleansing and building program can help treat allergies.
- Enzyme therapy along with amino acids can help cleanse the body of undigested protein and other toxins in the blood and cells.

Candida (candidiasis)

The overgrowth of the yeast organism *Candida albicans* is known as candidiasis. It debilitates the immune system. To get *Candida* under control, a person must adhere to a strict dietary regime. *Candida* is scientifically classified as a fungus. This fungus can cause thrush and vaginal infections, as well as spread to any part of the body that is weakened.

Candida multiplies and develops toxins which circulate in the bloodstream and causes all kinds of symptoms and illnesses as well as chemical reactions in the body. *Candida* can cause a person to gain weight and help prevent the body from losing the pounds it needs to eliminate. The book, *Back to Health,* by Dennis Remington, M.D., and Barbara Higa, R.D., says:

> Yeast toxins seem to interfere with sugar metabolism in several ways. Besides interfering with sugar absorption by the cells, several other steps in sugar metabolism are blocked. Normally, the sugar forms glucose — the major source of fuel for most body cells. This glucose can come directly from breakdown of various foods in your intestines, especially from sugars and carbohydrates. Proteins in the diet are broken down to amino acids, and amino acids can be converted into glucose by a process called gluconeogenesis (the making of new glucose). After the food from a meal has been completely digested and no further energy is available from that source, sugar stored in the form of glycogen (in the muscles and liver) can then be converted into glucose and used for fuel. About 2,000 calories of energy are available. Various protein tissues in the body, including muscle tissues, can also be readily broken down to glucose when energy is needed.
>
> These beautifully designed metabolic systems normally keep the blood sugar relatively constant, and provide a steady source of energy at all times. Yeast toxins may, however, interfere with the various enzyme systems which are responsible for mediating all these processes. If you can't effectively utilize your sugar stores, or break down your amino acids for fuel, then you must rely mainly on food

presently in the intestines. Between meals, there may be low blood sugar and excessive amounts of hunger, encouraging the ingestion of more food than your body can effectively waste, resulting in weight gain. As you experience this hunger, it will probably be for carbohydrates, and especially for refined sugars, since the sugars are the most readily available source of fuel.

Yeast toxins may also impair fat metabolism. As mentioned earlier, the higher insulin levels are responsible for producing excessive amounts of fats, that are stored in the fat cells. Insulin also interferes with the breakdown of fat stores. Fat is normally broken down into components called fatty acids and glycerol, which are further metabolized to produce energy.

Under normal circumstances, fatty acids are burned almost exclusively through muscle tissue. Special enzymes called beta-oxidation enzymes found in muscle cells are necessary in order to burn fatty acids. Very active people, especially endurance athletes, have large numbers of beta-oxidation enzymes, allowing them to burn large amounts of fat for fuel, while inactive people tend to have very few of these enzymes. Most overweight people are just not active enough to have good levels of fat-burning enzymes, and this is made even worse with candidiasis. There may also be an impairment of the enzyme systems responsible for deriving energy from fatty acid metabolism, thus further limiting the amounts of fats that can be used as fuel.

In a sense, these problems that interfere with fat metabolism could be compared to having huge piles of firewood stacked all around your house, a firm contract with someone who keeps bringing more, and only a very small stove in which to burn it . . .

Candida albicans can produce false estrogen and make the body think it has enough, signaling it to cease production. It also sends out messages to the thyroid making it think it has enough thyroxine, therefore stopping production. These results can cause menstrual irregularities and hypothyroid problems.

SYMPTOMS

- fatigue
- sore throat
- bad breath
- chronic infections
- thyroid problems
- panic attacks

- swollen glands
- digestive disorders
- constipation
- depression
- indigestion

CAUSES

The overuse of antibiotics is one of the main causes of candidiasis. Antibiotics are also found in beef, chicken, and dairy products. A high sugar diet encourages the *Candida* growth. Repeated pregnancies without time for the body to replenish nutritionally can also be a problem. Nutritional deficiencies, birth control pills, steroid hormones, and many drugs weaken the immune system and set the stage for *Candida* growth.

NATURAL TREATMENT AND DIETARY GUIDELINES

Yeast multiplies rapidly when starches and sugars are consumed. Eliminate sugar, white flour products, yeast breads, wine, beer, fruit juices, cheeses, mushrooms, vinegar products and limit fruit to small amounts. Hydrochloric acid and pancreatic enzymes help to prevent yeast overgrowth.

The liver is responsible for filtering the blood. When overloaded, it is difficult for it to eliminate the yeast growth. Clean the liver and the bowels, purify the blood, and stick to a diet rich in vegetables, millet, brown rice, buckwheat and other whole grains. Beans are high in protein. Nuts such as almonds are high in nutrients and protein. Avoid peanuts; they carry a cancer-causing mold called aflatoxin. Garlic has antifungal properties. A great juice drink can be made from carrots, celery, parsley, one clove of garlic and ginger. Fiber is important for cleansing the intestinal tract, as well as absorbing toxins.

Cleanse the blood, the lower bowels and improve digestion and liver function. Patience with diet will pay off in the long run.

NUTRITIONAL SUPPLEMENTS

Vitamin A is essential for healthy mucous membranes.

Vitamin C with bioflavonoids encourages healing and prevents infections.

B-complex Vitamins (yeast-free) are necessary for proper digestion and they also help the liver to eliminate toxins. Extra biotin, B6 and B12 are needed.

Vitamin E is an antioxidant for healthy veins and immune function.

Multi-vitamin Supplements will build up the immune system.

Iron is important for a healthy immune system and energy.

Multi-Mineral Supplements are necessary for proper function and utilization of vitamins.

Acidophilus is important for increasing friendly bacteria and digestion. It is best taken first thing in the morning or just before going to bed so it can reach the colon. Hydrochloric acid can destroy the effects of acidophilus.

Chlorophyll and Blue-green Algae will purify the blood and provide nutrients. They also help the body produce its own interferon.

Flaxseed Oil and Salmon Oil help strengthen the immune system.

Germanium and Co Q-10 improve oxygen supply to the arteries.

Cat's Claw (uña de gato) helps combat *Candida* infection throughout the entire body. It especially works on the intestinal tract.

Formulas that include the ingredients *Caprylic Acid, Pau d'Arco, Echinacea and Garlic* are useful for eradicating fungal infections in the body.

FACTS AT A GLANCE

- *Candida* yeast toxins can contribute to sudden weight gain and can hinder a person from losing unwanted pounds.
- *Candida* can contribute to fatigue by preventing the body from properly converting sugar into energy.
- *Candida* can cause many symptoms which can be mistaken for other diseases.

- *Candida* can interfere with function of the thyroid gland and the liver.
- Avoid yeast-containing foods and take supplements to cleanse the system of *Candida.*

Epstein Barr and Chronic Fatigue Syndrome

The Epstein Barr virus is a common organism that usually remains dormant in most people, unless the immune system is weakened. The virus also causes infectious mononucleosis, sometimes referred to as the "kissing disease." It often strikes young people.

EBS is chronic and can linger for months and maybe years before a person realizes what it is. Mononucleosis strikes all at once, hits hard and may last two to four weeks or longer if the diet isn't corrected.

Symptoms

- fatigue
- recurrent upper respiratory tract infections
- sore throat
- swollen lymph nodes
- memory loss
- aching joints and muscles
- low-grade fevers
- headaches
- night sweats
- poor concentration
- irritability
- deep depression

Causes

Stress has been implicated as a possible cause in that highly motivated people seem more prone to develop the disease. Other causes that have been linked to this disorder are mercury poisoning from amalgam fillings, hypoglycemia, anemia, hypothyroidism, sleep apnea, food and chemical allergies, weak adrenal function, parasitic infections, amino acid deficiencies and infection with the yeast *Candida albicans*. This fungus can prevent the body from utilizing sugars properly, blocking the body's energy production and causing extreme fatigue.

NATURAL TREATMENT

Rita Elkins, in her book *The Home Health Advisor*, makes several suggestions for dealing with fatigue. Very mild exercise will increase stamina and oxygenate cells. Exercise also helps to improve sleep. Exercise and massage, in combination with elevation of limbs, are believed to stimulate the lymphatic system, which can help strengthen the immune system.

Stay away from allergens. EBS victims are often more prone to allergic reactions since their immune systems are compromised. Talk to others who suffer from the disease and share your feelings with your family and friends.

DIETARY GUIDELINES

Foods to support the immune system include brown rice, whole grains such as buckwheat, millet, whole oats, rye, and yellow corn meal, fresh fruits and vegetables, sprouts, seeds, nut milks and vegetable juices. Cleansing the body with lemon water, chlorophyll, and vegetable broths will help heal and strengthen the body.

Most people with CFS/EBV also have *Candida*. A diet eliminating sugar, alcohol, mushrooms and all fungi, molds and yeast in any form, fermented foods such as sauerkraut, soy sauce, all dry roasted nuts, potato chips, soda pop, bacon, salt pork, lunch meats and cheeses of all kinds is recommended.

NUTRITIONAL SUPPLEMENTS

Vitamin A and beta-carotene build the immune system and stimulate interferon production.

B-complex Vitamins prevent fatigue and improve stamina and mental alertness.

Vitamin C with bioflavonoids protects against germs and viruses and heals the cell walls. It also supports adrenal function.

Vitamin E protects the cells from damage.

Acidophilus improves digestion, combats yeast infections, and helps the body manufacture B-vitamins in the intestinal tract.

Chlorophyll and Blue-green Algae help the body produce interferon for restoring health.

Co Q-10 and Germanium help oxygenate the cells to promote a healthy immune system.

Essential Fatty Acids (like evening primrose oil, flaxseed oil, salmon oil) help the body balance glandular function and improve vitality.

Digestive Enzymes are important keys to proper assimilation of nutrients to feed the cells, tissues and organs of the body.

Free-form Amino Acids are easily digested proteins to help heal the cells.

Single Herbs that help with CFS/EBV include: echinacea, garlic, goldenseal, pau d'arco, red clover, burdock, cat's claw and milk thistle.

FACTS AT A GLANCE

• Stress debilitates the immune system.
• Mild exercise helps relax the nervous system.
• Taking herbs supports the immune system.
• Detoxify the body of harmful elements so the body can cleanse and heal.

Lupus

Lupus is a chronic inflammatory disorder of the connective tissues and appears in two forms: discoid lupus erthematosus (DLE), which affects only the skin, and systemic lupus erythematosus (SLE), which generally affects other organs as well as the skin. It can be fatal and is characterized by remissions and flareups, like its cousin disease rheumatoid arthritis.

Corticosteroids are the main medical treatment for SLE. But there are no miracle drugs. It is a complex disease. Those who use natural methods of cure have been known to be able to stop using cortisone and other drugs within six months to a year. Lupus, as well as rheumatoid arthritis, are conditions which are difficult to move out of the body. Medical doctors and researchers believe that the increasing degenerative diseases we are suffering from are side effects from the many immunizations people have been given over the past few decades. These immunizations have the effect of making it impossible for our immune systems to know whether a substance in the body is its own or whether it comes form the outside of the body.

Symptoms

• non-deforming arthritis (joint pain and stiffness)
• "butterfly rash" and sensitivity to light
• aching
• malaise
• fatigue
• low-grade fevers
• chills
• weight loss
• possible lymph node enlargement, abdominal pain, nausea, vomiting, diarrhea and constipation
• heart and kidney problems, headaches, irritability and depression

Causes

There are three theories as to the cause of SLE. First, SLE is an abnormal reaction of the body to its own tissues, caused by a breakdown in the immune system. Second, certain factors may make a person more susceptible to SLE than others. Stress, streptococcal or viral infections, exposure to sunlight, immunizations, and pregnancy may all affect the development of the disease. Genetic predisposition is also suspected. And third, SLE may be aggravated by certain drugs, from anticonvulsants to penicillins to oral contraceptives.

Another cause is that protein molecules from dairy products (pasteurized and homogenized) can readily pass through the intestinal wall and form antigen antibody complexes which can cause arthritis and form the complexes of SLE. (In the past, only natural health practitioners believed this about dairy products, but this information comes from a reputable medical journal, *The Journal of Allergy and Clinical Immunology*). See reference on "Leaky Gut Syndrome."

NATURAL TREATMENT

Herbs, diet and other therapies would normally help move out toxic waste matter and mucus with other disorders, but not with SLE. The waste simply stirs around in the bloodstream, unable to be removed from the body. This is because the body's ability to remove accumulated waste is hindered and retarded by a constant buildup of parasites. Lack of parasites makes for easier cleansing.

A fast of water and juices can be used to great effect, as well as garlic, catnip and cayenne enemas. Mild exercise is beneficial. Taking blood purifiers with herbs that kill worms and parasites is suggested. Cleansing the bowels and liver are important.

Systemic lupus is a degenerative disease whose power and final outcome depend largely upon the mental, physical, emotional and spiritual attitude of the sufferer. Never give up, for the nature of a degenerative disease is that the body is in an unnatural and confused state. Correct that state, and healing will come.

DIETARY GUIDELINES

A change of diet is the first consideration, for the patient should not be putting good things into his body through the front door, while bringing garbage in the back. In addition to the natural treatment above, large amounts of naturally cleansing foods like raw vegetable and fruits juices, as well as a mild food diet, are the only ways to heal this disease. Enjoy foods such as endive, whole oats, lentils, beans, split peas, whole wheat, barley, brown rice, asparagus, green peas, sunflower seeds, broccoli, cabbage, brussels sprouts, almonds, avocados, buckwheat, millet, salmon, chickpeas, parsley, watercress; and green salads with lemon and olive oil dressing.

Avoid all white sugar and white flour products, meat, fried foods, stimulants such as alcohol, caffeine, tobacco, and all drugs, especially birth control pills, and antibiotics; any drugs will create more toxins and put a burden on the liver. Avoid taking too much salt.

NUTRITIONAL SUPPLEMENTS

Nervine herbs should be considered first. They are black cohosh, hops, lobelia, hops, lobelia, passion flower, skullcap, valerian, and willow bark.

Black Walnut and Goldenseal will kill parasites and worms.

Garlic, Aloe Vera and Burdock are blood cleansers.

Capsicum and Comfrey are healing to the skin and mucous membranes.

Dandelion helps to detoxify the liver. Devil's claw cleans deep in the cells.

Echinacea, Oregon Grape, and Pau d'Arco clean the blood and lymphatics.

Use a *liver cleansing combination* containing herbs like cascara sagrada, red clover, sheep sorrel, peach, barberry, echinacea, licorice, Oregon grape, stillingia, sarsaparilla, prickly ash, burdock, kelp, and rosemary.

Cat's Claw (uña de gato) cleanses the intestinal tract, assists the body's elimination of parasites and helps restore immune system function. (Note: as cat's claw is detoxifying the intestinal tract, excessive gas may result. This will diminish as the colon is cleansed.)

Black Walnut oxygenates the blood, which kills parasites. It is used to help balance blood sugar levels, and helps the body eliminate toxins and fatty materials.

FACTS AT A GLANCE

• Lupus is a chronic inflammatory disorder of the connective tissues.
• Lupus is a parasite-related disease.
• Avoid junk foods, and eat a nutritious diet high in raw foods.
• Take natural supplements; cat's claw is an especially important herb to take for lupus.

Section 8

The Nervous System

A wise man should consider that health is the greatest of human blessings, and learn how by his own thought to derive benefit from his illnesses.

HIPPOCRATES

The Body's Electrical Wiring

The central nervous system consists of the spinal cord and brain. The peripheral nervous system comprises the nerves that extend out from the spinal cord and the base of the brain to other parts of the body. The autonomic nervous system regulates function of the internal organs. The nervous system is a very delicate and vital part of the body and needs to be treated and fed properly. The central nervous system and the immune system are closely connected. When one system fails, the other is affected. The brain has the job of transmitting information back and forth from the immune system.

The brain is our most sensitive organ and reacts to poor nutrition, drugs, air pollution, junk food and impure water. When a brain neuron dies, it can never be replaced. The brain is vulnerable to lack of oxygen or glucose. It can be destroyed by drugs, alcohol and drugs together, concussion, stroke, toxic metals such as mercury and aluminum, and inflammation. Malnutrition during gestation and in early childhood causes irreparable damage to the structure of the brain.

Brain-starved infants lose their ability to develop properly. Alzheimer's disease creates a loss of memory, and autopsies on these individuals have disclosed extremely low brain levels of biochemical raw materials essential for synthesizing neurotransmitters, which helps make remembering and thinking possible. The lack of nutrients to the brain can cause serious problems with memory.

Brain and nervous system disturbances can start early in life and gradually increase. Researchers have found that dyslexia, learning problems, writing difficulties and other problems of the nervous system are connected with cerebral diseases. It may take years to manifest itself in a serious dementia disease, as it is a gradual process. Just because we all age doesn't mean we have to have memory and brain dysfunction.

As an interesting sidenote, medical doctors at the turn of the century published information linking the connection between the health of the colon and brain and nervous disorders. Many women with nervous disorders have had excellent success when they cleansed the intestinal tract with herbs and changed their diets.

Addictions

Whether it is sugar, chocolate, caffeine drinks, alcohol, tobacco or drugs, the number of women addicted to these substances is increasing. This silent epidemic is a major health problem in women and some seek help with antidepressants. Mind-altering drugs are very popular, and are increasing steadily in use. Addictions in women may show no outward signs to their family until there is a crisis and the addictive substance is taken away for a week or so. This causes severe withdrawal symptoms, such as fever, psychosis, and seizures from drugs such as heroin. Less addictive drugs can cause shakiness, loss of appetite, memory loss, concentration problems, muscle cramps, insomnia, anxiety, panic attacks and agitation. These symptoms can be misdiagnosed by a physician and then additional drugs are given, which only increases the addiction.

Coffee is "an approved drug," which many people do not realize. The caffeine is addicting and very irritating to several parts of the body. It causes indigestion and irritation to the kidneys. It also wears down the nervous system. The phosphorus in soft drinks can cause the loss of minerals, such as calcium.

When sugar, chocolate and caffeine are mixed, they seem especially addictive. Chocolate is a high source of caffeine. Chocolate is very high in fat, and since it is very bitter it must be mixed with sugar to make it palatable. There are a lot of women who admit they are "chocolate freaks." They do not realize they are involved with a drug. The same pattern is seen in those who consume coffee and cola drinks. An addiction becomes a problem when it takes up a vast amount of time, money and energy, and begins to control one's life.

When the substance becomes an obsession and you think about it all the time, plotting the next time you will indulge, you have an addiction. Also when the food causes negative reactions, such as bloating, indigestion, fatigue or other symptoms and they are ignored, you have an addiction. Lack of control, making excuses, and denial of the negative side-effects are signs of addictions.

Symptoms

• dependency on a substance, used frequently
• symptoms such as headaches, anxiety, agitation and and insomnia
  develop when the addiction is not satisfied
• weight gain or loss
• panic attacks
• depression
• personality changes

Causes

The main cause of addictions is nutrient deficiencies. When the body is lacking vitamins, minerals and amino acids, addictions can manifest themselves. When we are lacking nutrients, allergies can develop. It seems to be a vicious cycle; the substance that we are addicted to becomes an irritation or allergy to the body.

An addiction is increased when the cravings are stimulated and subsequently cause a loss of appetite. The addiction prevents eating a nutritional and health-building diet. Many women on drugs either lose their appetite or their appetite is increased and they put on more pounds, which makes them more depressed than ever. There may be underlying causes such as negative emotions, inability to cope with everyday problems, and feelings of unworthiness.

Natural Treatment

For a woman to become balanced spiritually, emotionally, mentally and physically, she needs to value herself enough to take charge of her health. Stress effects the body when it is congested through constipation or malnutrition.

A liver cleanse is essential to help the body eliminate toxins. Many drugs and substances such as caffeine, tobacco, and alcohol accumulate in the body. They will remain in the tissues until a cleanse eliminates them. Use an herbal liver formula which contains milk thistle. First thing in the morning, use juice of one whole lemon or lime in a cup of warm water and add a teaspoon of grated or capsuled ginger, 1/2 teaspoon fenugreek, 1/2 teaspoon licorice root, and one tablespoon of pure olive oil. It can be blended before drinking.

A fresh juice cleanse for a few days at a time will help the body eliminate toxic substances in the tissues and cells. Use mainly vegetable juices to began with (fruit juices will increase the cravings for sweets such as chocolate, and sugar.) Carrot, celery, endive, and parsley juice combined are very nourishing and cleansing.

Read all you can about addictions and what the side-effects are. Increasing knowledge of the harmful effects will give a better understanding and a greater will power to overcome any addiction. An exercise program will increase circulation and oxygen to the brain. Walking out of doors in the fresh air is very stimulating to the blood and brain.

Dietary Guidelines

A change of diet is essential for cleansing the tissues, colon, liver and cells. Addictive substances build up in the body and may take months to eliminate. Eliminate red meat, fast foods, sweets and white flour products from the diet. They not only are deficient in vitamins and minerals but contain substances that are harmful to the body.

Fasting is one of the best ways to eliminate toxins. Start slowly, like one day a week, then increase to two or three days at a time.

Use a lot of vegetables, both in fresh salads and steamed lightly. They are rich in minerals which will help to strengthen the body while eliminating the toxins. Green drinks are very nourishing and cleansing. Make a cup of juice by adding parsley, celery, endive, cucumbers, green leafy lettuce and wheatgrass. You can add carrot, apple or pineapple juice to the green drinks. Wheatgrass juice is purifying.

Substitute a grain drink such as Postum® or Pero® for coffee. Use whole grains instead of white flour products. Use herbal teas instead of black tea, especially relaxing teas, which will strengthen the nerves. Have a lot of pure fresh water handy; distilled water is very cleansing.

Digestive enzymes should be taken after eating and between meals, in order for undigested proteins in the cells to be broken down and eliminated. This will increase digestion and assimilation and increase the benefits of food eaten.

Use beans, nuts, seeds, and sprouts often, as they are packed with nutrients. Almonds are rich in calcium and magnesium. Soak them for twenty-four hours in pure water. They can be blended in water to make a milk or use in brown rice and millet dishes for more nutrients.

Nutritional Supplements.

B-complex Vitamins are very important to support the nervous system and help the liver to detoxify.

Antioxidant nutrients are essential: these include vitamins A, C, E and minerals selenium and zinc.

Multi-mineral Supplement are needed for every function of the body. Minerals and vitamins work together to restore health to the body.

Calcium and Magnesium are important to strengthen the nervous system. When the nerves are fed properly it is easier to cope with addictive problems. Some women crave chocolate around the time of their menstrual cycle and it is thought by some to indicate a magnesium deficiency.

Gymnema sylvestre and Chromium will help in digestion and assimilation and heal the pancreas.

Blue-green Algae and Chlorophyll will clean and nourish the blood. They will also speed the cleansing of toxins from the cells and blood.

Digestive Enzymes are essential for proper digestion and assimilation of food. They will also help the body eliminate particles of undigested protein which create toxins in the body.

Hydrochloric Acid is necessary for minerals to assimilate properly. It will also prevent toxins, viruses, germs, parasites and worms from invading the body.

Lecithin is needed to nourish the myelin sheath that protects the nerves.

Essential Fatty Acids are found in flaxseed oil, evening primrose oil, borage oil, black currant oil, and salmon oil. The glands need these nutrients in order to function, especially to produce enzymes and hormones.

Amino Acid supplements are important for healing and repairing the cells of the body.

Herbs for Cleansing are contained in red clover formulas. A combination of echinacea, licorice, peach bark, burdock, prickly ash, Oregon grape, sheep sorrel and as red clover will clean the blood and liver.

Formulas containing bioflavonoids, grapefruit pectin, milk thistle, and indoles will strengthen the immune system and contain nutrients to help heal the body.

Colon Cleanser is essential and should include cascara sagrada, rhubarb, goldenseal, barberry, lobelia, ginger and cayenne.

FACTS AT A GLANCE

• Addictions are common in women and lead to nutritional deficiency and antidepressant dependency.

- A positive approach and diet change is necessary.
- Fasting is one way to clean the blood and cells of addictive substances.
- Malnutrition is one cause of addictions. Healthy people seldom need addictive substances.

Anxiety, Panic Attacks and Phobias

Anxiety can trigger fear or panic attacks. When the brain is under stress, anxiety reactions can be triggered. People with phobias are often overwhelmed by mental, physical and emotional stress and cannot control anxiety.

Women become withdrawn, irritable, anxious, listless, and experience stresses unique to women alone. They menstruate, become pregnant, and go through menopause. They are the caretakers of aging parents and handicapped children, besides possibly handling stresses of divorced parents, or even their own divorce. Women who work have the added burden of handling household duties. Women feel these challenges of life more than men. We feel that one of the main reasons that women "feel" the pressures of daily stress more may be that a woman's liver is more sluggish and cannot eliminate excess estrogen. Excess estrogen builds up in the body and when the liver and colon cannot eliminate it properly, it backs up into the blood and can reach the brain and cause anxiety and other problems.

SYMPTOMS

- anxiety
- dizziness
- feelings of unreality or disassociation
- spaciness
- confusion
- a floating sensation
- feeling of claustrophobia when around crowds

CAUSES

Anxiety, panic attacks or phobias are directly related to the health of the nervous system. The brain and nervous system are connected. Lack of nutrients allows toxins to build up in the body. Minerals are especially necessary for a healthy nervous system. Minerals prevent toxic metals from accumulating.

Nervous system disorders are related to a toxic colon. It creates autointoxication, a way of self-poisoning the body. This causes irritants to wear down the nervous system and brain.

Sugar, soda pop, chocolate, white flour products and meat all take a toll on the body. These products contain no nutrients beneficial for health. In fact they pull essential nutrients out of the body, and if not replaced, will cause irritation to the nervous system.

When the body is prone to nervous disorders, look for body stressors such as *Candida,* food allergies, trace mineral deficiencies, hypoglycemia or female-related problems. Controlled studies at Yale University and the National Institute of Mental Health showed that the amount of caffeine in eight cups of coffee (also caffeine drinks), significantly increased anxiety in 15 of 21 panic-prone patients. The researchers theorize that caffeine blocks the function of adenosine, a substance which lessens the firing of nerve cells in certain brain areas.

NATURAL TREATMENT

Hypoglycemia is very common in those that have panic attacks. Changing to a diet conducive to treating hypoglycemia has helped many people. This condition is usually precipitated by a high-sugar and refined carbohydrate diet. It calls for a change of diet, eliminating sugar, caffeine, white flour products, heavy meat eating, while introducing more vegetables, grains, sprouts, beans, brown rice and millet, raw almonds, raw seeds, herbal teas and pure water to the diet. Stay away from even fruit juice for awhile, until the body become balanced again. Small amounts of fruit are fine.

Hypoglycemia can bring on symptoms of fatigue, depression, anxiety, irritability, confusion, and mood swings.

Drugs are not the answer to panic attacks or anxiety. They may provide relief at first, but the body builds up a tolerance to any drug. Actually, drugs can increase life's problems. Some people become so relaxed they lose all ambition to accomplish anything in life. You cannot think clearly under the influence of tranquilizers; they only interfere with the healing process of the body.

Panic attacks, anxiety, and phobias are real; they are very frightening to those who go through them. The problem needs to be faced. Learn not to let it frighten you, and realize that it will pass. Learn that with the proper nutritional approach you can overcome these feelings. Changing eating habits and adding supplements will help heal the brain and nervous system.

DIETARY GUIDELINES

Add a free-form amino acid supplement to the diet to begin. As you learn to use whole grains in your diet, they will provide the amino acids for nervous system disorders. It is well known that tryptophan is the precursor to the neurotransmitter serotonin, which relieves anxiety by soothing the nerves and increasing relaxation. Serotonin levels are found depleted in people who have anxiety problems. Histidine deficiency causes irritability, uncertainty, anxiety and mental confusion.

Glycine is another amino acid lacking in anxiety patients. It helps control our motor functions. The deficiency results in spacy feelings, and jerky, quick movements. The central nervous system needs large amounts of taurine.

Use brown rice and millet dishes. Cook half millet and half brown rice in your favorite dishes. They are high in B-vitamins, calcium and magnesium, which are essential for nervous system disorders.

NUTRITIONAL SUPPLEMENTS

Stress Formula should contain hops, skullcap and valerian, and schizandra to strengthen nerves. It should contain calcium and B-vitamins.

Digestive Enzymes are very beneficial in neurological disorders. A lack of enzymes can cause nervous system disorders. Enzymes will help break down the toxins causing irritation to the nervous system.

B-Vitamins are essential for healing the nervous system. Extra B12 and B6 will speed the healing.

Vitamins A, D, and E help in strengthening the immune system.

Vitamin C with bioflavonoids helps the body deal with stress and is essential for the formation of adrenal and thyroid hormones.

Multi-mineral Supplements are essential since all minerals are necessary for a healthy nervous system. They function by regulating functions of the muscular and nervous systems. Herbs have minerals that are easily absorbed. Alfalfa, kelp, horsetail, oatstraw, and almost all herbs are rich in minerals.

Magnesium levels that are low are seen in those with severe stress problems. It is the relaxer of the body.

Lecithin is high in choline and inositol, which are necessary for the health of the nerve sheath.

Essential Fatty Acids contain properties to reduce tension and anxiety. They help to stimulate prostaglandins, which relax muscles.

Herbs for Anxiety include skullcap, hops, chamomile, passion flower and valerian root. In clinical studies, St. John's wort has shown to positively alter brain chemistry, improve mood swings and help relieve depression.

Ginkgo, Gotu Kola and Suma increase circulation to the brain. They help in carrying nutrients to the brain area.

Ginger has an antispasmodic effect on the muscles.

Licorice Root nourishes the adrenal glands and helps the liver to eliminate excess estrogen.

Colon Cleanse is necessary for eliminating a buildup on the colon wall, which interferes with digestion and assimilation of nutrients. Use enemas, colonics or a special herbal formula to gradually peel off the crust on the colon. It should contain cascara sagrada, ginger, raspberry, barberry, lobelia, barberry or buckthorn, rhubarb, fennel and cayenne. This formula cleans and nourishes the colon to restore normal function.

Blood Cleanser is needed to help clean and eliminate toxins from the blood. It should contain red clover, burdock, buckthorn, sarsaparilla, licorice, prickly ash bark, barberry, peach bark, echinacea, sheep sorrel, and cascara bark.

Liver Herbal Formula is necessary for the liver to be cleaned and nourished, to be able to eliminate toxins. It should contain milk thistle, dandelion, yellow dock, bayberry, Oregon grape, lobelia, goldenseal, and red beet root.

FACTS AT A GLANCE

• Anxiety attacks are real.
• A sound nutritional approach will give long-range benefits.
• The nervous system can be destroyed by sugar, caffeine,white flour products and a high-meat diet.
• Herbs, vitamins, minerals and other supplements help in nourishing the nervous system.

Chemical Imbalance

A chemical imbalance is not a disease in itself, but is any condition which alters the normal pattern of chemical reactions in the body. This can take place prior to an illness. Depletion of nutrients experienced in bulimia can create an chemical imbalance in the body.

Many women are being diagnosed as having a chemical imbalance in the brain. It is seen as an illness that needs antidepressants in order to replace the natural chemicals that have reached low levels in the body. Drugs only cover up the symptoms; they will not give lasting results.

Nutrition is many times the answer to a chemical imbalance. In order to change the imbalances of the body, get rid of symptoms, and help the body heal itself, nutrients are the answer. Correct food, including vitamins, minerals and herbs will help the body heal itself. The brain is the seat of emotions and is another organ in the body. It needs to be nourished properly just as much as the heart, lungs, liver or any other part.

Anyone with a chemical imbalance usually either needs more nutrients than the average person, or they are not assimilating their nutrients. Because the brain is extremely sensitive it suffers when the body seems strong in other areas; consequently this condition will alter the functions of neurotransmitters.

There are three major neurotransmitters that appear to have a profound effect on the brain: acetylcholine, serotonin and epinephrine. These are made in the body but they require dietary biochemical precursors of these substances. What we lack in our diet causes an imbalance in these neurotransmitter.

Although the kinds of nutrients needed by all humans are the same, some people have a much larger requirement for certain vitamins and minerals in order to recover from their illness.

Symptoms

• emotional disturbances
• deep depression
• confusion
• irritability
• forgetfulness
• inablity to cope with everyday problems

Causes

Malnutrition, intestinal toxemia, and malabsorption are the main causes of a chemical imbalance. A congested colon and liver prevent food from digesting properly. Lack of the vital nutrients causes an imbalance in the body. White sugar and white flour, as well as soft drinks, caffeine, alcohol, and all refined food leech nutrients from the body. Diet plays a big part in creating an imbalance in the body. Even eating too much meat leeches minerals and can cause an imbalance.

Natural Treatment

The first thing we need to realize is that the health of the body is really up to the individual person. Research and study will help to understand how the body works, and what it needs to heal itself.

Correct nutrition will play an important role in recovering from any illness. Eating whole grains and more fruits and vegetables, instead of refined products, is helpful. Adding more raw food to the diet helps the body heal. Raw juices provide concentrated nutrients that will heal the body faster. Many people have gone on raw juice diets and healed themselves from heart disease, cancer, and many other diseases, simply because they gave their body what it needed to recover.

Exercise increases circulation and helps the body in the healing process. It provides oxygen, the most critical nutrient for health of the body. Oxygen metabolizes our food and turns it into energy. Oxygen can also destroy or neutralize free radicals. A positive attitude is very healing. Learning to think good thoughts, give more love and the ability to forgive are part of the healing process of the body.

DIETARY GUIDELINES

Cooking whole grains in a slow cooker or in a thermos overnight is one way to retain the B-complex vitamins and enzymes. Enzymes are essential for every function of the body. Mixing rye, whole oats, whole wheat, buckwheat and kamut together, and adding almonds and a few currants or dates makes a delicious breakfast.

Add more beans, peas and lentils to the diet. They can be added in soups, main dishes and in salads. They are high in protein and sulfur which help prevent cancer and eliminate heavy metals.

Grains are valuable and nourishing. Millet is a grain that is easy to digest. It can be mixed with white rice until you get used to it. Then add half millet and half brown rice. Grains are valuable and nourishing. Amaranth has more protein than wheat and contains vitamin C. Kamut is a newly discovered ancient grain, and is organically grown. It is high in protein, pantothenic acid, calcium, magnesium phosphorus and zinc. Quinoa is rich in calcium. One cup contains as much calcium as a quart of milk, and assimilates better than milk. Spelt is the most easily digested of all the grains. It is high in B-vitamins, iron and potassium and rich in fiber and protein. Grains will help balance body chemistry. They contain nutrients that will supply serotonin and melatonin in the brain.

Use vegetables freely. Salads and steamed vegetables are very nourishing. They go well with beans and grains. They make a complete meal. Use fruits in the season when they are rich in nutrients. They are best when tree-ripened.

NUTRITIONAL SUPPLEMENTS

Amino Acid Supplements are needed to help the healing of the mind. Diet alone may not provide this important brain stimulant. They should be taken on an empty stomach. Amino acids encourage production of the neurotransmitter epinephrine, which stimulates the brain and increases metabolism.

Vitamins A, D, C, E help protect the body from free radical damage. They work with minerals to balance body chemistry.

Digestive Enzymes are necessary for preventing autoimmune diseases. Lack of enzymes prevents cooked food from being properly digested. Enzyme supplements will help heal the body and break down undigested food in the cells and blood.

Lecithin contains choline, which boosts the neurotransmitter acetylcholine and is needed to stimulate memory and learning. B-vitamins also boost acetylcholine levels in the brain.

B-complex Vitamins are essential to enhance brain neurotransmitters. Supplements will speed healing.

Essential Fatty Acids include flaxseed oil, evening primrose oil, borage oil, salmon oil, and black currant oil. These are required for normal development of the brain and nervous system. They help make a group of chemicals in the body called prostaglandins, hormone-like chemicals that regulate many functions and activities of the body.

Multi-mineral Supplements are necessary for balancing body chemistry. Calcium, magnesium and chromium deficiency can lead to depression.

Blue-green Algae, Chlorophyll, Spirulina, and Chlorella are rich in protein. They are also rich in vitamins and minerals and are easily digested.

Bee Pollen is rich in protein and B-vitamins, especially B12. It is very important in overcoming depression and imbalances in the body.

Gotu Kola, Ginkgo, and Suma stimulate brain function.

Nervine Herbs, which include passion flower, hops, skullcap, chamomile, valerian root, and St. John's wort, are high in minerals and vitamins that stimulate serotonin production in the brain. They will strengthen and nourish the brain and nerves.

FACTS AT A GLANCE

• Chemical imbalances are real.
• Drugs help cover up the symptoms, but only add more toxins to the body.
• Grains and nervine herbs help the body produce neurotransmitters in the brain.
• The body needs to be cleaned to digest and assimilate nutrients.

Depression

Depression is a real concern in our modern society. There are so many stresses in everyday life. Just keeping up with life is enough of a challenge, but when a person has to face emotional and physical obstacles, it can be too much and depression can result. Everyone gets depressed at one time or another, and this is normal. However, if it does not go away within a reasonable length of time, and stays deep-rooted, the cause definitely needs to be explored.

SYMPTOMS

• feelings of hopelessness
• finding no joy in life
• wanting to sleep all of the time
• feeling tired after sleeping all night
• experiencing loneliness, even when around people
• dislike of self and others
• wanting to escape life and problems

Women especially seem to be prone to depression. This is partly due to the immense responsibilities of balancing work and family duties. This can put a big strain on wives and mothers, and prevent them from performing every-day tasks that are necessary in raising children and running a household. Strengthening the nervous system with nutrition can help the body cope with stressors that can precipitate depression.

CAUSES AND TREATMENT

There are many reasons for depression. Unresolved memories of abuse, or a traumatic experience such as divorce, can trigger feelings of depression. These issues need to be addressed with proper treatment, and counseling may be necessary, but nutrition can go a long way toward healing the mind and emotions.

The two main causes of depression in most women are nutritional deficiencies and autointoxication, which can cause an imbalance of hormones.

Manic depression, which causes extreme mood swings, can cause a lot of misery for the person suffering from it, as well as for their loved ones. When someone you love or someone you are acquainted with is manifesting symptoms of antisocial behavior, before you make an appointment with a psychiatrist, please examine their diet. Is it loaded with artificial additives, white sugar, and pastries? Does the person smoke, drink, or consume an inordinate amount of caffeine?

Some symptoms of mental disorders include loss of interest in school and work, changes in sleep patterns, withdrawal from society, irritability, panic attacks, sudden attacks of rage, and lack of enthusiasm for association with family and friends.

We are including here a true success story of a girl who overcame mental illness through nutrition. Heather was diagnosed as a manic depressive and a borderline schizophrenic. She was a lovely and delightful person. At age thirty she was hospitalized for a suicide attempt and her stomach was pumped. All her life she was plagued with mental problems, and her family members had the same disorder. She said that desires to commit suicide and panic attacks were a way of life for her. Heather was on all kinds of drug therapy, using lithium, Haldol® and Oxazepan®. She underwent psychiatric therapy two times a week, but nothing seemed to help.

Heather was introduced to a nutritional approach by a friend. With a complete cleansing program, using herbs to clean her blood and colon, she began to gain her sanity. She started slowly to change her diet. She used nervine herbs such as valerian, lady's slipper, passionflower, skullcap, hops, and wood betony. She was able to experience her first night of restful sleep. She felt her health improve immediately. She gave up her medications. Her attitude became positive, and she is now well and happy, helping others who suffer from depression.

Doctors routinely prescribe drugs to treat depression. However, there is much controversy over the merits versus their side-effects.

The debate surrounding SSRI drugs such as Prozac, Paxil, Zoloft, Lovan and Luvox is that while they raise the level of a certain type of serotonin, they lower another. There is also concern that these drugs act as nervous system stimulants, which can result in altering one's perception of reality and impairing judgment. Despite the conflict enveloping Prozac, many doctors stand by it as a highly effective drug in treating depression. This class of drugs is designed to raise brain levels of serotonin by inhibiting the process of serotonin re-uptake, thereby keeping levels elevated in brain cells. This process prevents serotonin from going into the bloodstream. As mentioned earlier, some experts are concerned with this unnatural build up of serotonin in the brain. They warn against a hormonal cascade effect, which can, in some individuals, prompt bizarre or destructive behavior." (*Depression and Natural Medicine*, Rita Elkins)

When the body is strengthened with proper nutrients, the brain can handle stressful situations. Whole grains, such as millet, brown rice, whole oats, rye, buckwheat and whole wheat contain the amino acid tryptophan, which is responsible for producing serotonin and melatonin in the brain. When these neurochemicals are lacking in the brain, it can cause depression of varying degrees. Sugar can deplete the body of B-complex vitamins and minerals, especially calcium and magnesium. These nutrients are especially crucial to balanced mental health.

You can eat all the good food you can stand and take all of the supplements you can handle, yet if your body does not absorb the nutrients, these nutrients will not do much good. The keys to proper.

absorption are detoxification and digestion. Digestive enzymes will help the body process the nutrients from food and maximize its assimilation.

At the turn of the 20th century, Dr. J. A. Stucky, M.D., made the observation that the blood is poisoned through absorption of toxic material from the intestinal canal more frequently than from any other source.

The overproduction of estrogen in the body has been linked to autointoxication. When the body is loaded with toxins, the liver will be burdened and will not be able to process the excess estrogen. If the intestinal tract is not able to eliminate this estrogen, it is reabsorbed into the bloodstream and carried to various parts of the body, including the brain.

Autointoxication

For detailed information on this subject, please refer to the section on autointoxication on page 32 of this book, and read Louise Tenney's *Nutritional Guide with Food Combining*. An excerpt from the chapter on autointoxication says:

> Hippocrates claimed that chronic disease came from autointoxication, i.e., self-poisoning due to constipation. The deposits of accumulated waste in the colon release toxins which inflame the nerves, producing rheumatism, neuralgia, melancholia, hysteria, eczema, acne, headaches, and many other health problems. Hippocrates also taught the way to handle diseases: "Let food be thy medicine. . . ." Health experts believe that all sickness begins in the colon . . . Faulty digestion also plays a role in autointoxication. If food is not digested properly, amino acids can be converted by the microbes into powerful toxic substances (such as phenol, indol, indican, etc.). These can cause symptoms such as fatigue, nervousness, gastrointestinal upsets, skin problems, headaches, insomnia, glandular and circulatory system disturbances, etc.

Autointoxication also affects the functioning of both liver and brain. It will poison them via the bloodstream and can cause many problems; among them are poor memory, personality changes, and lower immunity. Autointoxication has also been linked to arthritis, breast disease and emotional disorders. Mental illness can be caused by this condition, especially constipation throughout the intestinal tract.

Dietary Guidelines

A high-fiber diet which is also rich in cruciferous vegetables is essential for balancing hormone levels. Eating foods rich in complex carbohydrates (brown rice, millet, buckwheat, whole wheat, oats, etc.) will help depression because they contain tryptophan, which has a calming effect. Turkey, fish and beans are excellent sources of protein, instead of red meat. Red meat has a constipating effect. Fresh or steamed vegetables will supply many essential minerals, as will essential fatty acids, bee pollen, and blue-green algae.

Nutritional Supplements

Single herbs include *Ginkgo biloba*, gotu kola, siberian ginseng, red clover, skullcap, and chamomile.

Herbal Combinations contain blood purifying formulas, skeletal system formulas, digestive enzymes, immune formulas, lower bowel combinations, nerve and stress formulations.

Vitamins and Minerals beneficial for depression include B-complex, calcium, magnesium, and multi-minerals.

Facts at a Glance

- Depression has many symptoms, but only a few basic causes.
- The main reasons for depression are autointoxication and a diet devoid of nutrients.
- When the body is strengthened with proper nutrition, the nervous system is able to tolerate more stress.
- Eat a high-fiber diet rich in complex carbohydrates and fresh or steamed vegetables.
- Take key nutritional supplements to help nourish the nervous system.

Insomnia

Despite all the changes a woman experiences in her lifetime, she is always supposed to remain sexy and attractive, to be assertive but not overly aggressive in a so-called man's world. She is also expected to hold down a full-time job but not to neglect their family.

It is no wonder that women can develop insomnia. Insomnia is a major problem in the United States. As many as ten million people suffer from severe insomnia. An occasional night of insomnia is common, but when it goes on night after night, something must be done. Medication for insomnia only treats the symptoms and does not get to the root cause.

The primary drugs used for insomnia are antihistamines and benzodiazepines. The antihistamines can be bought at drug stores. They act to prevent the manufacture of histamine in the brain. This will produce drowsiness and the ability to fall asleep. Insomnia drugs depress the central nervous system. Eventually they wear away the protective sheath which is the lining of the nerves and cause deterioration of the nervous system. They act upon the cerebral centers and interfere with the passage of impulses in the brain. Drugs depress brain function, and in large doses depress the brain centers responsible for maintaining the rhythm of respiration. Tolerance to these drugs often build up rapidly, leading to addiction and the need for higher and higher doses to produce the desired effect. The brain quickly adjusts to the presence of sleeping drugs so they are made ineffective.

If you wake up refreshed, you then know that you have had adequate sleep. If you wake up groggy, dull-headed and have to struggle to stay awake during the day, you have not had enough sleep.

SYMPTOMS

• unable to fall asleep
• wakeful periods during the night
• waking up in the night and unable to fall back to sleep

Causes

Certain diseases can cause insomnia, but the main causes are autointoxication and nutritional deficiencies. Lack of certain vitamins and minerals are linked with insomnia. For example B-complex vitamin deficiencies can cause insomnia. Supplemental B12 and B6 have helped people with long-standing insomnia. B6 assists in the formation of serotonin in the brain, and the B-vitamins also help the liver to eliminate toxins such as the excess estrogen. Certain minerals help in the metabolism of vitamins. Copper, calcium, magnesium, manganese, potassium and zinc are essential for all body functions.

Stimulants, like caffeine drinks, and drugs such as Anacin®, Excedrin®, Midol®, and Vanquish®, (among many others) cause the brain to become active if taken close to bedtime.

Alcohol and sugar overwork the liver and cause congestion. They also deplete the body of minerals. Sugar needs minerals for metabolism, and therefore robs the body of stored minerals.

Aspartame (found in NutraSweet® and Equal®) is a sugar substitute. It is found in diet drinks, diet foods, ice cream and yogurt, gum, pudding, and even encouraged for diabetics. Aspartame has been known to cause side-effects. The contents include the amino acid phenylalanine, aspartic acid and methanol (wood alcohol). Excessive amounts of methanol, a brain poison, can cause insomnia along with other side effects. Anxiety, stress, worry, and nervous tension can cause lack of sleep.

Natural Treatment

Exercise is important in allowing the body to become physically tired and produce a natural sleep. Walking in fresh air is very stimulating and provides oxygen to the lungs and brain. A mini-trampoline produces good exercise for the lungs and lymphatics without injury to the joints.

Use cotton sheets and cotton clothing to sleep in. They help the body to breathe better. The skin is constantly eliminating toxins, and synthetically manufactured clothing stifles the skin.

The colon and liver need to be cleansed and nourished. The large intestine can accumulate glue-like material that adheres to the walls and prevents nutrients from being assimilated and digested. The small intestine can collect mucus and toxins that can be re-absorbed into the bloodstream. These poisons can travel to the brain and cause insomnia.

Anxiety, stress, worry, and nervous tension can cause lack of sleep. Dealing with deep emotional problems will help the mind rest. Learn to eliminate suppressed anger, hate, bad feelings and any others that impede the healing of the body and mind.

DIETARY GUIDELINES

A good colon cleanse uses herbs that not only clean but help to rebuild a lazy colon. Herbs that act as herbal food for the small and large intestine are cascara sagrada bark, barberry, Turkey rhubarb root, red raspberry leaves, ginger, goldenseal root, lobelia, fennel, and cayenne.

The liver is the body's detoxifier and needs to be kept in good working order. Emotional imbalance is seen when the liver is congested. Herbs for the liver are: milk thistle, dandelion root, red beet root, goldenseal root, yellow dock, bayberry, Oregon grape root, kelp, and lobelia.

A good liver cleanse is useful first thing in the morning and includes a cup of hot water, juice of one lemon or lime, one teaspoon of pure olive oil, one half teaspoon of fresh ginger, one teaspoon of fenugreek and one half teaspoon of licorice root. This can be mixed in the blender.

Juice fasting is an excellent way to restore emotional health and prevent insomnia. A combination of endive, carrot, celery and parsley juice is beneficial.

Millet is rich in calcium and magnesium and is easy to digest. Start cooking it with rice first and then use half brown rice and half millet. Grains will help the body produce tryptophan which stimulates serotonin and melatonin in the brain. Use thermos cooking for complete nutritional benefits. You can use the grains for breakfast, in salads or in casseroles. They are tasty and very nutritious. Grains also add more fiber to the diet and help prevent colon congestion. Use more steamed vegetables and raw salads in the diet.

NUTRITIONAL SUPPLEMENTS

B-Complex Vitamins with extra B12 and B6 will help the body produce serotonin in the brain and helps the liver to detoxify.

Vitamin and Mineral Complex is necessary for the assimilation of all nutrients.

Vitamin C with bioflavonoids are needed every day, since the body cannot produce its own vitamin C. It helps feed the small capillaries, so nutrients can nourish the brain.

Digestive Enzymes are very essential for the digestion of cooked food as well as digesting protein build-up in the cells and the blood. They also break up the protein coating on viruses, germs and parasites.

Amino Acid supplements, with extra DL-phenylalanine, tyrosine, and methionine, help supply the body with neurotransmitters to protect emotional health.

Nervine Herbs will help strengthen, soothe and nourish the nervous system. These are black cohosh, blue vervain, catnip, chamomile, hops, lady's slipper, lemon balm, lobelia, passion flower, skullcap, St. John's wort, valerian root, and wood betony. They can be taken in capsules or in extract form.

Essential Fatty Acids are vital for every function of the body. They feed and nourish the cells and glands. They are found in flaxseeds, borage oil, black currant oil, evening primrose oil, and salmon oil. Women need these oils to balance weight and glandular function.

Lecithin is essential for nourishing the myelin sheath that protects the nerves.

Blue-green Algae is nourishing and cleansing to the blood.

FACTS AT A GLANCE

- Chronic insomnia can lower the resistance of the immune system.
- Diet change can strengthen the nervous system.
- Certain drugs, alcohol, caffeine and aspartame can cause insomnia.
- Supplements will help build up the nervous system.

Meniere's Syndrome (Tinnitus)

Tinnitus is commonly known as ringing or buzzing in the ears. It is very prevalent in the United States, with over 30 million people suffering from this condition. It is with them, more or less, all the time — a constant buzzing or ringing that never goes away. It can affect one ear or both. Both men and women can suffer from tinnitus, which strikes the young as well as the old. The hearing (auditory) nerve is closely connected with the nerve leading from the balancing mechanism located in the innermost portion of the ear (the labyrinth). Disturbances of the labyrinth may cause so much ringing in the ears that it can cause hearing impairment.

Symptoms

- ringing in the ears
- loss of hearing
- loss of balance
- nausea
- vomiting

Causes

A junk food diet can cause "plugged-up" ears. Mucus-forming foods can cause an accumulation of material in the head area and especially the ears. The head area requires more nutrition and circulation than any other single body organ. Poor nutrition causes clogged up blood vessels that help support ears and hearing. This happens over a period of years with gradual clogging up of the tubes to the ears. That's why we see so many elderly people with hearing problems. It is not only the elderly that are having hearing problems; we are seeing more and more children and even newborn babies with hearing problems. A factor causing hearing loss in our youth is noise pollution. Our ears are not meant to be exposed to loud noises for long periods of time. Nerve damage is an inevitable result.

Some other causes of hearing loss are fetal damage, trauma at birth, infections, drugs (people have complained after being treated with drugs [quinine is one example]), thyroid disease, diabetes, injuries, noise exposure, nerve deterioration and malnutrition. We have to realize that lack of nutrients can contribute to hearing loss. Dr. Paul Yanick, Jr., a clinical audiologist and holistic health expert says that tinnitus can be caused by ear wax accumulation, glandular problems, high blood pressure, aspirin, quinine or other commonly prescribed drugs. Exercise, a change of diet and learning stress reduction has helped tinnitus. Vitamin B6, niacin, pantothenic acid, vitamin E, choline and lecithin have also helped.

Natural Treatment

Dietary change is the most important thing you can do to help change the inner health. Mucus-forming food is the cause of most hearing problems and infections in small children. This can build up throughout the years and cause other ear problems. Herbal tinctures in the ears have helped many people. This helps to get circulation in the head area, as well as supplying essential nutrients.

Grape juice and green drinks are high in potassium. High potassium prevents autointoxication and a buildup of mucus in the ears. Smoking, alcohol, caffeine, and a high-meat diet are harmful. Exposure to cigarette smoke in the household can cause chronic middle-ear disease, as well as other problems in children. Smoke is dangerous for children who have lung and nasal congestion. Ear damage increases six-fold in children who grow up with passive smoke intake.

Diana is a mother of four children and is thirty-five years old. She has suffered from tinnitus off and on for years, even as a young girl. Her sister Sharon and her mother both suffer with this constant ringing in the ears. Diana noticed that when she is sick, the tinnitus is always with her. She also suffers with hypoglycemia, PMS and *Candida albicans*. Sometimes the ringing in the ears would last as long as a week; sometimes it would last a month and there were times it stayed with her for six months at a time.

Diana told her different doctors about the ringing in the ears, but they had no answers or suggestions of what could be done to correct it. In fact, most doctors just ignored this problem because she had so many things wrong with her. Nothing she took would stop it. At times it would stop on its own, but when she was on tranquilizers or sleeping pills it never stopped. In desperation one day she tried putting cotton in her ears, but it only made it worse. Nothing she did would stop the high-pitched ring in her ears.

As mentioned earlier, Diana had been battling candidiasis for years. She had a standing prescription at the drug store. It never gave her any permanent results. She finally realized that if she was going to battle this problem it would have to be done by herself. She completely changed her diet. While she was fighting her *Candida* problem, her tinnitus disappeared, never to return. The first thing she realized was that her digestion was seriously troubled, so she started taking enzymes for digestion along with acidophilus and aloe vera juice. She completely eliminated meat from her diet because of an immediate reaction with a headache, stomach pain and gas that lasted for hours. Giving meat up was easy for her because she was also giving up the pain, indigestion and the embarrassment. Diana went off milk, white sugar, white flour, and soda pop and started drinking herbal tea twice a day. Chamomile, alfalfa and red clover were at the top of her list. She added many fresh fruit and vegetables, grains such as millet, buckwheat, raw seeds and nuts, sprouts, beans, lentils and all wholesome and live foods.

There is much evidence from many parts of the country to support Diana's theory that her problem was nutritional. Nutritional deficiencies contribute significantly to most hearing-related problems, including tinnitus. A clean colon will assure that nutrients will be absorbed. The colon is where essential minerals and nutrients are taken by the blood and deposited in the tissues. Cleansing diets, juice fasts, herbal colon cleanses and colonic therapy will promote colon health. This will help dissolve mucus and eliminate toxins from the body. Herbal blood and liver cleansers are beneficial. Increased circulation through exercise, diet and supplements will provide lymphatic drainage and a healthy bloodstream.

DIETARY GUIDELINES

Eat a natural diet high in whole grains, fresh vegetables, fruits, nuts, seeds, sprouts, legumes, and beans. Enjoy almonds, baked potatoes with skin, apples, apricots (dried), cashews, sunflower seeds, black cherries, broccoli, carrots, dates, dried figs, leaf lettuce, lentils, dried beans, and whole grains (thermos cooked). Avoid fried foods and white flour and white sugar products.

NUTRITIONAL SUPPLEMENTS

There is evidence to support that herbal combinations have been very beneficial to ear problems such as tinnitus. Many kinds of ear problems have been helped with herbs. The head area needs a constant flow of nutrition for healthy ears, eyes and brain. Circulation in the ear area is very important, along with a change in eating habits. It is important to feed the nerves in the area at the base of the skull. The herbal extract combination to help provide circulation and nutrition is found in *Today's Herbal Health,* by Louise Tenney. This combination is healing to the motor nerves and should be used in both ears, even though one ear is involved. It can renew the motor nerves and related function in the ears. This combination, along with oil of garlic, can be beneficial in tinnitus problems. It should always be remembered that if there is a broken ear drum, you should wait until it is healed before anything is put in the ear. A fomentation can be used on the outside of the ear.

Chickweed contains antiseptic properties. It acts as a blood cleanser and helps to dissolve any material in the ears that would hinder healing. It strengthens and nourishes the inner ear area.

Black Cohosh helps increase circulation in the head area for proper healing. It is a nervine herb that strengthens and rebuilds the nervous system.

Goldenseal increases the tonic properties of the other herbs in this combination. It contains natural antibiotic properties to help stop infections.

Lobelia is an excellent herb for the nerves. It acts as an antispasmodic. It is one of the greatest healers in the herbal kingdom. It can be used for any illness with excellent results.

Skullcap helps to rebuild and nourish the spinal cord. The base of the skull is where the motor nerve is and when this nerve is congested skullcap will help.

Licorice contains glycosides which eliminates built-up mucus from the ear area. It has a stimulating action and will heal inflammations.

Ginkgo biloba improves memory and mental alertness by increasing circulation in the head area and supplying nutrients. It helps to reduce anxiety, tension, dizziness, headaches and symptoms of senility and age-related cerebral disorders. Studies have shown ginkgo to be very effective in helping eliminate tinnitus in test subjects.

Gotu Kola is a brain food. It helps balance the right and left hemispheres of the brain. It rebuilds energy reserves and stamina. It also helps to combat stress and helps improve reflexes. The nutrients in gotu kola are essential for the nerves as well as the brain.

Ginseng stimulates the entire body to overcome stress, fatigue and weakness. It stimulates and improves brain cells. It is used to normalize blood pressure, reduce blood cholesterol and prevent arteriosclerosis. It is said to improve vision and hearing.

Bugleweed equalizes circulation and helps in varicose veins. It strengthens the small capillaries for ears, eyes and brain health. It helps in all circulatory problems.

Suma balances circulation and helps to combat fatigue. It nourishes the brain and head area.

FACTS AT A GLANCE

• Disturbances of the labyrinth part of the ear may cause so much ringing that it can cause hearing impairment.
• A factor causing hearing loss in our youth is noise pollution.
• Lack of nutrients can contribute to hearing problems.

Migraine Headaches

Females suffer from migraine headaches twice as often as males. The tendency to get them also runs in families. It has been said that Napoleon suffered early in his life with migraine headaches. He was also affected with chronic constipation.

Migraine headaches develop when an artery in the head dilates. It throbs and the vessel wall expands, which causes pain. The spasms that develop can cause dizziness, ringing in the ears, seeing sparks or colors through the eyes and tingling in the temples.

Migraine headaches in women are linked with menstrual cycles. The Chinese see pain as an obstruction of energy flow. Migraines develop when the body is under a great stress or before the menstrual period when energy flow is slowed down. During the week before the menstrual cycle an imbalance of hormones takes place. This puts the liver in the position of detoxification and elimination.

The liver has a connection to the eyes. Migraine headaches usually start with changes in the eyes, such as pain behind or above one eye, or vision changes. Headaches seem to be related to toxicity which causes inflammation of the nervous system, and tightens up the muscles, which causes pain.

Symptoms

- pain above the eyes
- sensitivity to light
- throbbing pain in the temples
- changes in vision and/or seeing colors
- intense pain relieved by vomiting

Causes

Migraine headaches can be triggered by certain chemicals in food, or from alcohol, chocolate, cheese, caffeine drinks, hormonal changes, and stress. The main cause is toxins in the blood traveling to different parts of the body and causing congestion in those areas.

Autointoxication is the main cause of headaches. Migraines are sometimes called "sick headaches", which are relieved by vomiting. This stems from the stomach, where bile loses its powers, and undigested food causes toxins to be released. The endocrine glands attempt to direct the toxins to other eliminative organs. This hyperfunction can cause these organs to swell. As the pituitary gland enlarges it presses against its body enclosure, sometimes causing the severe pain of migraine headache.

Chronic migraine headaches are seen in people with leaky gut syndrome. Enzymes are essential for digesting food and preventing particles of undigested food to accumulate in the blood and cause irritations in different parts of the body. Thus allergies can develop in any part of the body.

The spine can become malpositioned or subluxed, which can pinch the nerves and cause pain associated with migraine headaches.

Other causes include drugs, lack of magnesium, blood impurity, acidosis condition, vitamin A deficiency, too much sodium chloride, anemia, fevers, food allergies, TMJ, eye problems, and a poorly nourished spinal cord.

Natural Treatment

The first step should be a detoxification program. This would include a colon, liver and blood cleansing. A kidney herbal formula will help eliminate acids from the blood. Herbal formulas are excellent for this. A change of diet is necessary in order to balance the chemistry of the body.

Exercise is beneficial in a detoxification program. Walking in fresh air will help provide more oxygen to the blood. Get some exercise at least three times a week.

Massage shoulder blades, the neck and back of head, all over head like shampoo. For migraines, massage the earlobes. Use a foot bath, alternating hot and cold water. Apply clay on the nape of the neck and forehead. Compresses are soothing on the nerves. Place a hot compress on the back of neck, while at the same time you place a cold one on the forehead. This will relax and stimulate at the same time.

Positive thoughts and loving feelings will help the body heal. Since stress triggers migraines, mental and emotional changes need to be made. Suppressed anger needs to be dealt with. Coming to grips with anger or hate and eliminating it from the body is a way to relieve stress.

DIETARY GUIDELINES

A hypoglycemia diet would be beneficial. Low blood sugar levels can trigger migraines. A positive diet change is important to cleanse the body. Eliminating the bad foods, such as sugar, white flour products, white rice, pasta, alcohol, caffeine, chocolate, and heavy meat diet, will take a burden off the body.

Start with eliminating one food at a time. Start with red meat and sugar. If you can do this for a month, you will never have the same taste for that food as you did before.

Add new foods one at a time. Start with brown rice and millet dishes. They will nourish and strengthen the nerves, because of the B-vitamins and calcium and magnesium content. Use almonds, which are rich in calcium, protein and other nutrients. Soak the almonds overnight, making them easier to digest.

Use avocados, which are rich in protein, vitamin A and essential fatty acids. Use fresh and steamed vegetables daily. A magnesium-rich juice drink can be made from carrots, celery, clove garlic, parsley, and a bunch of endive.

NUTRITIONAL SUPPLEMENTS

Digestive Enzymes help to break up the undigested protein in the blood and cells. Use after meals and in between meals.

Hormone Balancing Herbal Formula should contain *Vitex,* false unicorn, black cohosh, blue cohosh, licorice, cramp bark, red raspberry, ginger, and blessed thistle.

Vitamins A, C, E, Selenium and Zinc prevent free-radical damage to the capillaries in the head area.

B-complex Vitamins are necessary for proper nerve function. They help eliminate toxins from the liver.

Bee Pollen is rich in nutrients to help in hormone balance.

Cruciferous Vegetable Concentrate helps prevent toxin build-up and prevent accumulation of bad estrogen.

Feverfew is found to decrease the frequency of migraine headaches and lessen the severity of attacks.

St. John's Wort strengthens the nervous system. It also helps eliminate depression, headaches, insomnia and dizziness.

Glandular Formula includes licorice, kelp, dandelion, alfalfa, and wild yam.

Mineral Formula, consisting of extra calcium and magnesium, relaxes and strengthens the nervous system.

Stress Formula, including bee pollen, ginkgo, Siberian ginseng, capsicum, and suma, is very good for coping with stress and stengthening the nervous system.

Nerve System Formula, which consists of valerian, hops, wood betony, skullcap, black cohosh, mistletoe, lobelia, capsicum, and lady's slipper, works great for the nervous system.

Essential Fatty Acids are needed for brain function and help eliminate toxins from the capillaries. Examples include evening primrose oil, borage, salmon oil, flaxseed oil, and black currant oil.

FACTS AT A GLANCE

• Toxic colon and stomach are the main causes of migraines.
• Adding digestive enzymes will help in breaking up undigested food in the blood and cells.
• Eliminating caffeine products will help with migraines.
• Herbal formulas will help balance hormones.
• Changing the diet and adding supplements will help balance hormones and eliminate the cause of headaches.

Section 9

The Structural System

If we supply the conditions for health, health will follow with unerring certainty; but if the conditions are for disease, disease will sooner or later follow as the Law of Adjustment will permit.

ANONYMOUS

The Body's Framework

The body's structural system is comprised of bones, muscles and connective tissue. Bones provide support to the body and protection to vital organs. Inside each bone a bone marrow factory busily produces red blood cells. Bone is vital, living material which requires constant nourishment to keep it strong. It is constantly being renewed — breaking down, growing and regenerating itself.

Most of a woman's bone mass is acquired by age 30. At this point in life, twenty-five percent of her bone weight is water, 25 percent is a form of connective tissue called collagen, and 50 percent is calcium phosphate. The 200 bones of the body represent about 15 percent of the entire body's weight.

Ligaments, tendons and cartilage make up the connective tissue in the body. They help hold the bones together and to give it flexibility and movement. Minerals are vital nutrients for a healthy structural system. Calcium is the most prevalent mineral in the human body. Most of it is found in bones, and about two percent is contained in cells, the blood and soft tissues of the body. Other nutrients that the structural system requires include boron, vitamin D, magnesium and manganese. Glucosamine is another nutritional substance that helps the structural system by assisting the body in regenerating cartilage, especially in the joints. Muscles are an important component of the structural system. Properly functioning muscles allow movement of the body parts and organs. They are comprised of fibrous tissue that is able to contract and expand.

Arthritis

Arthritis is a debilitating condition that strikes old and young alike. It is a disease of the joints that involves pain, swelling, and sometimes deformities. The two most common types are osteoarthritis and rheumatoid arthritis. It can cause much agony and suffering to those afflicted. Those who suffer are looking for answers. The medical community does not seem to have all the answers. In fact, in many cases they say the cause is unknown. The forms of treatment include pain and inflammation reduction, physical therapy and surgery to replace joints in severe cases. Conventional treatments may relieve pain, but generally do nothing to alter the arthritis.

SYMPTOMS

- early morning stiffness
- joint swelling
- recurring tenderness in one or more joints
- unexplained weight loss
- redness or a feeling of warmth in joints
- fever

Osteoarthritis is the most common type of arthritis and often afflicts the elderly. It is more prevalent in women. It involves the gradual deterioration of the cartilage which can cause uneven wear between the joints, causing pain and stiffness. The most common afflicted areas are the hips, knees and spine. By the age of 80 almost 90 percent of individuals suffer from some degree of osteoarthritis.

Rheumatoid arthritis is a chronic destructive disease of the collagen and connective tissues. It can cause deformities and is characterized by inflammation and swelling of the joints. It usually first appears between the ages of 36 and 50 years of age, and is most often found in women. It can come and go in waves, almost disappearing and then recurring with marked intensity. The onset of rheumatoid arthritis can be heralded by fatigue, weakness, poor appetite, low-grade fever, and anemia.

CAUSES

Damp weather does not cause arthritis, but can aggravate the symptoms. Arthritis has been linked to glandular imbalances, a poor immune system, inherited tendencies toward the condition, or as a side effect from another illness or infection. Injury, surgery, prolonged overuse of the joints (excessive mobility) as in sports, deterioration of the joints associated with the normal process of aging, and biochemical changes in the body have also be implicated as causes.

Rheumatoid arthritis is considered to be an autoimmune disorder, where the body actually thinks its own tissues, especially cartilage, are foreign and attacks them. This sets up a painful, inflammatory condition which can result in deformity of the joints. It can also lead to destruction in other body areas such as the lungs, liver, kidneys, heart, and lymph nodes. Standard treatment with anti-inflammatory steroid-based preparations such as Prednisone can weaken the bone structure through demineralization and cause severe cases of osteoporosis. Nonsteroidal anti-inflammatory drugs such as ibuprofen, tolectin and others can destroy the body's cartilage cushion between the joints and slow down the body's natural ability to produce more. This can actually accelerate progression of arthritis.

There is a theory that parasites may be involved in this type of arthritis. In the book, *Guess What Came to Dinner,* by Ann Louise Gittleman, she says that a certain parasite called *Endolimax nana* is an amoeba cousin and "is a relatively new member of the bad-guy group of Protozoa, according to some researchers. It is the smallest of the intestinal amoebas, and the most convincing research of its underestimated virulence comes from Roger Wyburn-Mason, M.D., Ph.D., a British researcher who wrote *The Causation of Rheumatoid Disease and Many Human Cancers: A New Concept in Medicine.* Mason's book suggests that *Endolimax nana* is the cause of rheumatoid arthritis and a whole host of collagen-related diseases. This amoeba also lives in the lower bowel and can travel to other parts of the body . . ." His theory matches those of others who think that foreign organisms may cause rheumatoid arthritis by stimulating the body's reaction against the wastes and toxins they give off as they breed in the connective tissues and intestinal tract, causing an autoimmune reaction. Rheumatoid arthritis has also been linked to leaky gut syndrome.

Arthritis, like most diseases, has basic underlying causes. The body can only take so much abuse. When the systemic derangement and biochemical and metabolic disorders brought on by prolonged physical and mental stresses take over, then diseases invade the body. Faulty nutritional patterns, continual overeating, overindulgence in protein and the inability to digest them all weaken the body. These factors cause nutritional deficiencies, sluggish metabolism and retention of toxic wastes. It is no wonder diseases invade the body!

Natural Treatment

Warm baths and compresses may help alleviate pain. The active ingredient in cayenne pepper, called capsacain, has been included in many pain-relief ointments which are marketed today. Applied on the affected areas, many people say it is a great help. Gentle stretching exercises may be beneficial. Being overweight can contribute to arthritis by putting a strain on the joints of the body. Weight-loss can then be another positive measure to help the bones and joints stay healthy. Relaxation and stress management are important.

DIETARY GUIDELINES

Some doctors feel that arthritis may be related to food allergies. Prime suspects include members of the nightshade family, such as green peppers, tomatoes, and potatoes. Avoid red meat; it causes uric acid buildup in the body that can create sharp crystals to irritate the joints. This leads to an arthritis-related condition known as gout. Steamed carrots, celery and cabbage are nutritious. Eat cold-water fish such as salmon. They contain Omega-3 fatty acids which have anti-inflammatory properties. Omega-6 fatty acids, found primarily in plant sources, also benefit those with arthritis. Some people have been successful on vegetable diets and herbs. White flour, white sugar, coffee, cola drinks, alcohol, fried foods, pork, fats and heated oils and salt-loaded food is detrimental to those with arthritis.

NUTRITIONAL SUPPLEMENTS

Essential fatty acids can be very beneficial in treating the pain caused by different forms of arthritis. The following information was published in the March 1994 issue of *Prevention Magazine:*

A study conducted at the University of Pennsylvania following rheumatoid arthritis patients gives hope for relief from the pain accompanying the condition. Gamma-linolenic acid (GLA), which is an Omega-6 fatty acid found in evening primrose oil and borage seed oil was used in the study. The patients were given either a daily dose of 1.4 grams of GLA or cottonseed oil which has no GLA. After six months of the therapy, the group receiving the GLA had less pain and swelling of the joints than the other group. More research is being done to understand the value of GLA.

A related Danish study using 51 patients with rheumatoid arthritis also showed promise for Omega-3 fatty acids. The patients were put on a 12-week program of either Omega-3 polyunsaturated fatty acids or a typical fat composition of the average Danish diet. There was significant improvement in the pain and joint stiffness in the fish oil users. The article was published in the *European Journal of Clinical Investigation,* October 1992.

Dr. Joel M. Kremer, M.D., head of the division of rheumatology at the Albany Medical College, says that it may take three to four months for benefits to occur. He says, "It appears that fish oil provides an alternative building block for molecules that participate in the inflammatory process. The end products formed from fish oil have beneficial effects on dampening inflammation and, perhaps, some elements of the immune response associated with disease. Fish oil may also affect the way cells in the body signal each other."

Glucosamine is a vital nutrient which helps the body produce cartilage and synovial fluid. This is especially important as a person ages and their natural ability to replace cartilage in the joints decreases. Glucosamine can boost the body's ability to create new cartilage.

Alfalfa helps neutralize acid in the body, and contains a form of calcium which is easily assimilated by the body. Alfalfa is rich in minerals.

Devil's Claw has been shown to have healing powers in arthritis, rheumatism, diabetes, arteriosclerosis, and liver, kidney and bladder diseases.

Manganese is a mineral known to be essential for cartilage regeneration.

Vitamins A and C, Pantothenic Acid, Folic Acid and Zinc are all important for the body's production of cartilage.

Calcium and Magnesium work together to promote strong bones.

Histadine is an amino acid with anti-inflammatory properties that can reduce pain and swelling. It is also involved in tissue growth and repair.

Methionine is an essential amino acid that is crucial for the creation of cartilage. It also has natural anti-inflammatory abilities.

Burdock reduces swelling and uric acid deposits in joints and knuckles. It is an excellent blood cleanser.

Bromelain reduces inflammation and swelling. It also relieves tension pain and helps dissolve dead cells.

Yucca is a cleansing agent and contains plant nutrients that act like cortisone in the body without the side effects. It promotes healing and enhances the absorption of nutrients.

Cat's Claw (uña de gato) has strong anti-inflammatory properties and has shown to help arthritis and many autoimmune disorders.

FACTS AT A GLANCE

- Arthritis can be caused by many factors, including poor diet.
- Key supplements, like glucosamine, essential fatty acids and devil's claw, among many others, have shown to naturally relieve arthritis symptoms without side-effects.
- Osteoarthritis is caused by deterioration of cartilage which normally cushions the joints.
- Rheumatoid arthritis is an autoimmune disorder that primarily afflicts women.

Muscle Disorders

Muscle cramps (spasms) can be caused by nutritional deficiencies such as a loss of major minerals which act as electrolytes. Any condition that purges the body of fluids (vomiting, diarrhea, use of diuretics) can cause electrolyte depletion. Muscle spasms can develop by lifting heavy objects improperly and straining the muscles during sports activities. However, there are specific muscle disorders that require more extensive treatment. They include the disorders described below.

Fibromyalgia and Fribrositis

The following information on fibromyalgia is found in *The Complete Home Health Advisor,* by Rita Elkins:

Most people have never heard of the term "fibromyalgia" and unfortunately, even some physicians are not familiar with the disorder. If you have suffered the unexplained muscle aches that are typical of the disease, you have have gone from doctor to doctor looking for answers. Fibromyalgia is one of the most common disorders seen by rheumatologists, and yet it is probably one of the least familiar and understood conditions. Victims of this disorder, mostly women, are often unaware that they are suffering from a specific ailment. Fibromyalgia belongs to a family of disorders that are characterized by an overreaction to what is considered a normal stimulus. Some of these also include insomnia, irritable bowel syndrome, and migraine headaches.

Not too long ago, this particular disorder was considered to be a psychosomatic illness, which was particularly troubling to its victims. Fibromyalgia is another in a long line of disorders that is considered to be a by-product of Western lifestyle and is rarely seen in underdeveloped countries.

SYMPTOMS

- *Physical:* Fibromyalgia typically causes sore shoulders, hips, neck and back muscles, an inability to sleep well or non-restful sleep, persistent fatigue, and tenderness in the elbows and knees. Fibromyalgia can be very bothersome and create in its victims a feeling of discouragement and frustration. Frequently, victims of this disorder assume they must have some form of arthritis.
- *Psychological:* Unless you find a physician who is familiar with this disorder, your symptoms may be considered psychosomatic.

CAUSES

While the specific causes of this disorder are unknown, EEG tests showed that victims of fibromyalgia had a specific type of disruption in their brain wave patterns while they were asleep. The meaning of this brain abnormality as it relates to the disease remains inconclusive. Other possible causes include tension, viral infections, trauma, unusual exertion, nutritional deficiencies, and in rare instances, thyroid disease.

Fibrositis

Fibrositis is a condition characterized by stiffness and joint or muscle pain, accompanied by muscle and fibrous connective tissue inflammation. There are similar symptoms and causes among all sufferers. And there are techniques available to alleviate the pain.

Fibrositis is a syndrome. It is composed of several symptoms and goes by different names, including muscular rheumatism and fibromyositis. Fibrositis is diagnosed only after the pain has been present for at least three months and often years. The only apparent problem upon medical examination is the presence of tender points in different muscles and in areas where tendons join the bone. Seventy-five percent of sufferers are women. The majority who have fibrositis are between the ages of twenty and fifty.

SYMPTOMS

- anxiety
- severe headaches
- exhaustion
- irritable bowels
- joint pain
- nervousness
- sensitivity to humidity

Although these symptoms are not uncommon in the general population, they are found with much higher frequency in patients with fibrositis. Recognizing this association alerts us to some important clues, one of which is that if we look at fibrositis as a purely muscular problem, our view of this disorder is going to be far too narrow.

CAUSES

Trying to pinpoint the cause of fibrositis is often difficult. It seems to be triggered by a number of conditions which start with a susceptibility on the part of the sufferer. The causes appear to be numerous and involve environment, body and mind. The onset of this condition may come following a climate change, infection, or physical or emotional trauma. It may go into remission and then recur, becoming chronic. A major stress — whether physical, such as an automobile accident with injury, or emotional, as a death of a loved one or the loss of a job — can bring on the symptoms. Among fibrositis sufferers the causes vary, but the symptoms are often similar.

Natural Treatment, Dietary Guidelines and Supplements

Avoid red meats, fatty foods and acidic foods such as tomatoes and vinegar.

Acidic Foods can interfere with the body's absorption of calcium, which can cause muscle spasms.

Drink plenty of fluids, especially freshly-squeezed vegetable and fruit juices.

Carrot Juice is highly recommended. Eat plenty of green leafy vegetables.

Kelp and Chlorophyl supplements are also recommended.

Calcium and Magnesium are very important for proper muscle contraction and nerve function and should be taken as a supplement daily. Magnesium in particular has been shown to help ease the symptoms of fibromyalgia. A calcium deficiency can actually cause muscle cramping. Good sources of dietary calcium are yogurt, skim milk, and low-fat cheeses. In the case of fibromyalgia, calcium/magnesium supplements may be more effective. Magnesium increases the body's absorption of calcium. Taking a calcium/magnesium supplement at bedtime may help reduce pain and promote sleep.

Potassium is vital to proper muscle functioning and, like calcium, can cause muscle pain if levels get too low. Potatoes, bananas, dried peaches and prunes are good natural sources of potassium. If you exert your muscles routinely, take a potassium supplement.

Silicon also helps promote calcium absorption.

Vitamin E improves overall circulation. A deficiency of vitamin E has been linked to muscular aches and cramping.

Hops is considered a tonic for the nerves and a natural tranquilizer.

Lobelia helps to calm and soothe the nerves and helps with sleep difficulties.

Saffron helps with the normal digestion of fats.

Safflower contains linolenic acid, which helps with the assimilation of fats.

Skullcap and Valerian calm the nerves.

Cat's Claw (uña de gato) has shown to help alleviate the pain and inflammation of muscle disorders, particularly fibromyalgia.

Rest, Heat and Massage help alleviate discomfort. *Chronic Muscle Pain Syndrome*, by Paul Davidson, M.D., outlines some methods of treatment known as the Retrain Program, most of which have to do with relaxation techniques.

Education: Learn about the disorder and do something about the problem.

Muscle Training: This includes muscle stretching and fitness. Massage can help relieve muscle pain and stiffness for short periods of time.

Stress Control: Learn to control the stress in your life. Discuss the things that bother you with a close friend. This can help put problems in perspective. Do not overcommit yourself. Set priorities and limit commitments on your time.

Carpal Tunnel Syndrome

Even though carpal tunnel syndrome is not specifically a muscle disorder, it is included in this section because of the pain and inflammation it inflicts in the hands and wrist. The following information was taken from *The Complete Home Health Advisor,* by Rita Elkins:

> In the age of the computer keyboard, carpal tunnel syndrome has become somewhat of a liability of fast typing for extended periods of time. This kind of stress on the wrist can create pressure on the nerve by overworking the tendons, which makes them swell.
>
> Carpal tunnel syndrome develops over months or usually years, and is the result of continued repetition of movements of the hands or wrists. It involves damage to the nerve which carries brain signals between the brain and the hands. This median nerve, which passes through the carpal tunnel created by the wrist bones, can become crowded when tissues in the tunnel become inflamed. Carpal tunnel syndrome is a fairly common disorder, particularly for middle-aged women. It can affect one or both of the hands.

Symptoms

- *Physical:* Carpal tunnel syndrome can cause a tingling sensation in the thumb or other fingers; numbness of the thumb, middle or index finger; inability to perform tasks requiring dexterity; and shooting pains that go into the fingers or up into the forearm. If you have carpal tunnel syndrome, your little finger will not be affected. Tapping the wrist may also cause you to feel a tingly feeling. The pain and tingling of this disorder may increase during the night, especially if the wrists are bent. Frequently, by simply shaking the hand or rubbing it, the symptoms of carpal tunnel syndrome may temporarily stop. Remember that chronic pain located in any joint could be a symptom of arthritis.

Natural Treatment, Dietary Guidelines and Supplements

Very mild hand exercises such as rotating the wrists in circles helps to increase circulation and may alleviate some of the tingling. Exercise should be used with caution, as resting the wrists is sometimes more effective to control symptoms.

Cold packs may help to relieve swelling.

Change the position of your hands when crocheting, knitting, typing, holding tools, etc. to encourage better circulation. Use handles, pencils, pens, curling irons, scissors, etc. that are large and easy to operate. Also, it is not uncommon for people to sleep with their wrists bent against the mattress, which can aggravate symptoms of carpal tunnel syndrome. Before going to bed, use a wrist splint to keep your wrist straight, which takes stress off the nerves. These splints, which are usually made of metal with Velcro® fasteners, can be purchased at medical supply sources or can be especially made to fit your hand by a physical therapist.

Use a hand rest specifically designed for your typewriter or computer keyboard.

Use your whole hand when holding onto an object. If doing a manual job that involves a repetitive movement, take a break from the activity every 30 minutes.

A low-fat diet, which inhibits fatty deposits, is thought to be beneficial for carpal tunnel syndrome sufferers. Foods to emphasize are brown rice, whole grains, lentils, sunflower seeds, salmon, tuna, avocados, turkey and fresh fruits and vegetables. Avoid high-fat foods, smoking, stress and caffeine. Avoid the excessive consumption of protein, which studies have linked to a predisposition to carpal tunnel syndrome.

Vitamin B6 has shown to help relieve nerve-related disorders. There has been some conjecture that a lack of B6 can actually cause carpal tunnel syndrome. Dosages should be discussed with a health-oriented doctor. Improvement is usually not seen for at least a month to six weeks.

Vitamins A, C, D and E are all vital to tissue repair and healing, and can contribute to reducing inflammation. Vitamin C plays a significant role in connective tissue regeneration.

Calcium and Magnesium help calm the nerves and keep the nervous system healthy and functioning.

Potassium is important in proper nervous system function and in controlling the body's water balance.

Chromium and Zinc facilitate tissue healing.

Turmeric is a natural anti-inflammatory herb which can be applied as a paste to the affected area to help control pain and swelling.

Ginkgo biloba improves circulation, which can help to decrease tendon and tissue swelling.

Hawthorne Berry helps clean the veins of unwanted deposits.

Bromelain is an enzyme that should be taken for its ability to lessen swelling and inflammation.

Cat's Claw (uña de gato) has shown to help alleviate inflammatory muscle disorders, and helps cleanse the entire intestinal tract of toxins.

FACTS AT A GLANCE

• Inflammatory disorders respond, in part, to rest, heat and massage. In cases of initial swelling, as in carpal tunnel syndrome, a cold pack may help.

- Learn to control stress in your life.
- Avoid acidic foods.
- Take key supplements of herbs, vitamins and minerals.

Osteoporosis

We do not like to think of ourselves as "falling apart," but when the condition known as osteoporosis sets in, this is what happens. As women age, and the production of estrogen diminishes, the calcium, which needs estrogen to be metabolized is not taken into the bones, and gradual loss of bone tissue through the process of demineralization occurs. However, younger women who don't menstruate because of stress or not eating (anorexia) are more susceptible to osteoporosis because of diminished estrogen production.

SYMPTOMS

- muscle cramps, especially in the legs and feet at night
- tiredness and nervousness
- bone pain, especially in the lower back
- premature gray hair
- heart problems and high blood pressure
- periodontal (teeth and gum) disease
- loss of height

Bones require a wide range of balanced minerals for bone strength and density. Calcium needs to work as a team with proper ratios of other minerals, especially phosphorus, magnesium, manganese, boron, silicon and zinc, as well as vitamins C and D. If these are not present in the diet in sufficient quantities and balance, then the calcium will not be assimilated properly. Indeed, it may even deposit in soft tissue areas and cause bone spurs, kidney stones and arthritis-like symptoms.

CAUSES

Soft drinks contain phosphoric acid, which provides excess phosphorus. This upsets the mineral balance in the body, and prevents calcium and other important minerals from being assimilated by the body. One study quoted in the *Journal of Nutrition* demonstrated that female athletes consuming carbonated drinks experienced 2.3 times more fractures than those who didn't drink them (118 [1988]:657-660).

Caffeine consumption over a period of time may cause loss of bone mass because it causes the body to eliminate excessive amounts of calcium via the urinary tract.

Sugar: The urinary secretions of zinc, calcium and sodium are increased when the diet is high in sugar. This causes severe mineral imbalances. In addition, when calcium is taken at the same time as sugar, the body will not absorb the calcium.

Chocolate, like sugar, inhibits the body from absorbing calcium and other vital minerals.

Salt, especially in excessive amounts, can significantly increase urinary secretion of calcium. In one study, 200 mg of salt per day was fine, but 2,000 mg caused a high rate of calcium excretion. Ailsa Goulding, Ph.D., of the University of Otago in New Zealand, found that when young women added a teaspoon of table salt to their daily diets, the amount of calcium loss greatly increased. This amount of excreted calcium was calculated to potentially diminish bone mass by approximately one-and-a-half percent per year.

Aluminum can be absorbed and thereby accumulate in bones. This can reduce the creation of new bone and hasten the percentage of bone breakdown (resorption). This increases the chances for osteoporosis. Dietary sources of aluminum include fluoride-containing products, aluminum beverage cans, antacids, baking powder, aluminum cookware, processed cheeses and pickles. Note that eating citric acid products (or anything with the word "citrate" taken at the same time as an aluminum-containing substance) greatly enhances the body's absorption of aluminum. The body can also take in aluminum through the skin from antiperspirants.

Excess protein: Consuming a high-animal protein diet can promote loss of calcium from the bones. The body takes calcium from the bones in order to counteract the acidic by-products of protein breakdown, and then the calcium is excreted from the body via the urinary tract.

NATURAL TREATMENT

Weight-bearing exercise enhances bone remodeling (the breakdown and rebuilding of bone tissues). It increases bone mass and density. A weight-bearing exercise is that in which pressure is put on a bone by the body's own weight or through the force of a muscle contracting against it. Examples of weight-bearing exercises include walking, hiking, climbing, jogging, running, bicycling, jumping rope, aerobics, dancing and tennis. This type of "stress" especially strengthens bones.

DIETARY GUIDELINES

Eat a diet rich in whole grains, especially buckwheat and brown rice, which contain high amounts of magnesium and silica. Other foods rich in vital minerals include the grain millet, green leafy vegetables, almonds, soybeans, sesame seeds, lima beans, and red and white beans.

NUTRITIONAL SUPPLEMENTS

Phosphorus, in approximately a two-to-one ratio to calcium, contributes to the hardness of bones. (If the diet is consistently high in phosphorus and protein and low in calcium, dangerous loss of bone mass can take place because of mineral imbalance.)

Magnesium, Calcium and Phosphorus work together as a team to ensure strong bones.

Manganese is essential for normal bone growth and calcification. Research indicates that lack of manganese can contribute to the thinning of bones.

Boron: Research at the United States Department of Agriculture indicates that boron works similarly to estrogen in post-menopausal women to prevent demineralization of bone. Boron increased the blood concentrations of estrogen, in the same percentages as that of women who were taking regular estrogen replacement therapy. In addition, it was found that boron reduced the loss of calcium through the kidneys by 44 percent.

Silicon plays a major role in promoting healthy bones. It is thought that it is especially needed in the early stages of bone development. Research shows that animals placed on a silicon-deficient diet developed bone defects.

Zinc helps regenerate new bone tissue. Zinc works with vitamin D to help calcium absorb into bone tissue. Low zinc levels have been found in the blood and bone tissues of elderly people with osteoporosis (Atik, O.S. 1983. "Zinc and Senile Osteoporosis." J. Am. *Geriatr Soc* 31:790-791).

Vitamin C: Animal studies indicate that lack of vitamin C can contribute to osteoporosis by reducing bone formation and increasing the rate of bone resorption (breakdown of old or damaged bone tissue, resulting in loss of bone mass). Vitamin C also helps strengthen the structural proteins of bone tissue.

Vitamin D helps contribute to the absorption and deposition of calcium in bone tissue. The bones can become "soft" if the diet is low in this nutrient. The bones actually bend, instead of maintaining their normal strength. In children, this condition is known as rickets; in adults it is called osteomalacia.

Alfalfa helps the body assimilate many nutrients, especially calcium and protein. It contains high amounts of calcium and is rich in trace minerals. It provides phosphorus, iron, potassium and eight essential enzymes.

Kelp provides all minerals known to stimulate health. It provides both major (macro) and minor (micro) minerals, also called "trace" minerals.

Oatstraw is rich in silicon and calcium, and provides the building blocks for new bone growth.

Horsetail is considered one of the best for supplying silica (silicon) to promote the proper healing and regeneration of bone tissue.

Comfrey is a traditional herb used in wound healing. Comfrey expedites the process of strengthening and mending bone tissues. It is especially high in calcium, potassium, and phosphorus. It is also high in vitamins C and A.

Facts at a Glance

- Osteoporosis is the cause of 90 percent of all fractures after the age of 65.
- The average American woman loses one-and-a-half inches of height each decade after menopause as a result of vertebral collapse.
- Osteoporosis is the most common systemic bone disorder in the United States. It affects 15 million people, primarily women, causing thousands of injuries and deaths per year.
- Over $1 billion a year is spent on treating conditions related to osteoporosis.

(The above facts were taken from *Healthy Bones: What You Should Know About Osteoporosis,* by Nancy Appleton, Ph.D.)

Section 10

The Integumentary System

Beauty is a pledge of the possible conformity between the soul and nature, and consequently a ground of faith in the supremacy of the good.

GEORGE SANTAYANA

The Billboard of Health

The health of the hair, nails and skin is an indication of the overall health of the entire body. When the skin has eruptions, rashes, and allergic reactions, it means the inner skin or mucous membranes also have eruptions. The skin is the largest elimination organ. The scalp also eliminates constantly.

Lack of essential minerals is also a cause of hair loss and unhealthy skin. Any disease that impairs the vitality of the body has an effect upon the hair and skin. Hair loss and problems with the scalp and skin are symptoms of an imbalance within the body.

The hair and skin need to be treated internally and externally. The proper shampoo, without chemicals and harsh detergents, is the first line of defense. Loss or discoloration of the hair is generally due to the lack of hair building elements in the blood or to sluggish circulation in the scalp. Many experts advise shampooing daily to remove dirt and impurities from the environment. Also, toxins are eliminated constantly through the skin and the scalp. Massaging the scalp before washing will help to loosen up dead skin and increase circulation.

The skin needs natural ingredients in its cleansers and moisturizers to ensure that the pores are clean and free from dirt and other toxins for healthy looking skin. Diet has a profound effect on the health of the skin and hair. The blood needs nourishment through vitamins, minerals, fresh food, and herbs, which are beneficial to healthy hair and skin. The hair and nails also need protein and minerals.

Acne is probably the leading skin disease. Teenagers and young adults account for the largest number of skin patients. Other skin disorders are skin cancer, warts, fungal infections and psoriasis.

The nails can also mirror the health of the body. White spots can indicate a lack of minerals or poor assimilation of nutrients. Ridges going lengthwise can indicate anemia or having had anemia in the past. It could also be a lack of B-vitamins and adequate protein. Iron supplements containing yellow dock and dandelion would help in the assimilation of iron. Bulging or too flat nails mean a diet change is needed. Pink nails indicate good circulation.

Brittle nails that break in layers may indicate a deficiency of B-vitamins, iron or silica. Splitting nails may be due to lack of hydrochloric acid. Horizontal ridges may reflect a deficiency of protein, calcium, silica or sulphur. It could also stem from illness or severe stress, which could cause a deficiency of B-complex vitamins.

Hair, Fingernail and Skin Disorders

Hair, nails and skin health depend on the shampoos and conditioners we use for the hair and the cleansers we use for our skin. Vitamins, minerals, amino acids and enzymes are important for the health of the hair, nails and skin.

There are many toxic chemicals that can damage the hair and skin by absorption through the skin. Mineral oil, propylene glycol, lye and formaldehyde, along with many other chemicals, are used in hair and skin care products. These ingredients are not allowed in food but are permitted in commercial hair and skin products.

The health of the skin depend on the health of the kidneys and colon. The skin is considered the third kidney. When the colon is congested it backs up into the kidneys, and when the kidneys are congested, the skin takes over to attempt to protect the body by eliminating toxins.

SYMPTOMS

• balding, dry, brittle and dull hair
• ridges in the nails, easily broken, thin and dry, and brittle nails
• blemishes, wrinkles, acne, blackheads, and overall dull skin

CAUSES

Hair problems are caused by hormonal imbalance, hyperthyroidism, nutritional deficiencies, stress, disease, X-ray therapy, anesthesia, drugs, drastic reducing diets, pesticide poisoning, and glandular imbalance. Birth control pills can alter normal hair growth and rob the body of vitamin A, folic acid, magnesium, zinc and other nutrients.

During menopause the hormonal balance causes radical changes in the hair, scalp and skin if a nutritional diet is lacking. Unwanted hair on the face is usally due to overproduction of male hormones in the body. Nutritional deficiencies and a congested colon can cause an imbalance in hormones. Nail problems are caused by mineral and vitamin deficiencies, anemia, lack of protein and illness.

The skin is the largest organ of the body. It has two functions: one is to protect the delicate tissues from being exposed to dirt, bacteria, and air pollutants; and the second is to eliminate toxins to be disposed through the kidneys and colon.

NATURAL TREATMENT

Exercising in the morning to the point of sweating, then skin brushing followed by a warm shower or bath will stimulate hair and skin health. Try this and you will have more energy.

Use only natural products to clean and nourish the hair and skin. Tea tree oil shampoo help clean the dead cells and dandruff from the hair, and leave the hair fresh and conditioned.

Boils and blemishes are examples of a need for internal cleaning. A change of diet and an increase in water intake frequently can eliminate these problems. However, if you drink and bathe in chlorinated water, it will absorb in the body and age the skin.

Avoid refined sugar foods, hydrogenated oil, ham, bacon, hot dogs, corned beef, lunch meat, alcohol, tobacco, processed food, fried foods and too much salt. Preservatives and rancid oils retard hair growth and plug up the skin. These all deplete nutrients and enzymes from the body. Salt retains waste in the tissues and helps create conditions such as blemishes and dandruff.

Treat your nails to a manicure by soaking them in a mixture of warm water, a mild cleanser and a few drops of olive oil and vitamin E. Then push the cuticles back gently with a soft towel. Massage your nails with olive oil and vitamin E again. File the nails in one direction only; using a sawing motion weakens the nails. Buffing the nails stimulates circulation and promotes growth.

DIETARY GUIDELINES

A clean colon and digestive system help to prevent poisons from accumulating. Juice fasting and colon cleansing will help in the digestion and assimilation of nutrients that are essential for healthy hair, nails and skin.

Amino acid supplements will help nourish the hair, nails and skin. The nails are about 95 percent protein. Carrot and celery juice will supply vitamin A, calcium and other nutrients for the health of the integumentary system.

Millet is high in protein, calcium and magnesium and is easy to digest and will nourish the body. Brown rice is high in B-complex vitamins, especially if cooked slowly, to retain its nutrients.

NUTRITIONAL SUPPLEMENTS

Vitamin A (beta-carotene) is necessary for healthy hair, nails and skin. It helps in new cell growth. It prevents dry, flaky scalp, and dry, brittle hair. It protects the skin from aging, blemishes and becoming thick and dry.

B-complex Vitamins aid in tissue growth, control oil gland secretions, combat dandruff, speed healing, aid in moisture absorption, mend split ends, help prevent hair loss and increase circulation. B12 and B6 are anti-stress nutrients and prevent dry, dull and lifeless hair. A lack of folic acid can cause hair, eyebrows and eyelashes to fall out. PABA, biotin, folic acid and pantothenic acid assist gray hair to regain its normal color.

Essential Fatty Acids help keep the hair lustrous and the skin clean and healthy. They are found in the following oils: evening primrose, flaxseed, borage and black currant.

Lecithin is vital for health of the hair and creates thick and shining hair. It is also good for the skin and nails.

Blue-green Algae and Chlorophyll are rich in vitamins and minerals, especially vitamin K.

Minerals are essential for healthy hair, nails and skin. Copper works with iron and zinc to help the hair retain its natural color.

Digestive Enzymes are essential to assure the nutrients will be digested and assimilated.

Jojoba promotes hair growth and helps remove accumulated cholesterol from the scalp so that the new hair follicles can emerge unimpeded. Kelp is rich in minerals and works with vitamin E for assimilation. It also prevents dry, brittle, fading and falling hair.

Oatstraw and Horsetail are rich in silicon and trace minerals for healthy hair, nails and skin. Silicon helps in the assimilation of calcium.

Sage is an astringent and acts as a scalp tonic. It helps stimulate hair growth.

Yarrow stimulates, cleanses and tightens pores in the head to prevent hair loss. It also helps in regulating liver function, which is necessary for healthy hair.

FACTS AT A GLANCE

- Health of the colon and kidneys determine the health of the skin and hair.
- Vitamins and minerals enhance the health of the skin, hair and nails.
- Poor nutrition can cause unhealthy hair, nails and skin.
- Exercise increases circulation and healthy hair, nails and skin.
- Eliminating a bad diet and increasing the consumption of nutritious foods help nutritionally benefit hair, nails and skin.

Section 11

Special Interests

*Look round the habitable world: how few know their
own good, or knowing it, pursue.*

JUVENAL

This "Special Interest" section deals with issues unique to and
deserving the special attention of today's woman, such as the harm
that sugar can do to the body, modern-day concerns such as breast
implants and toxic shock syndrome, and other topics. We hope that
you will find this section very informative and enlightening.

Herbs Especially for Women

BEE POLLEN

Bee pollen is considered a complete food. It is rich in vitamins,
minerals, amino acids and enzymes. It is a great supplement for
women to boost stamina, endurance, and brain function. It strengthens the immune system, circulation and aids in digestion with its

enzyme content. It prevents the onset of addictions by strengthening the whole body.

Bee pollen helps in pregnancy and produces rich milk for the infant. It aids menstrual problems and menopausal symptoms. It stimulates sexual function by balancing hormones. It can help protect against cancer.

BILLBERRY (*Vaccinium myrtillus*)

Bilberry is beneficial for strengthening the capillaries and small veins. It is helpful with varicose veins, which are common during pregnancy and will also help protect from blood clots. Bilberry strengthens the eyes and helps protect from strokes, heart attacks and blindness.

BLACK COHOSH (*Cimicifuga racemosa*)

Black cohosh helps balance hormones, especially estrogen and progesterone. It strengthens the uterus and is useful for irregular or scanty menstruation, helping diminish muscular aches and pains. It helps with menopause symptoms, and when used in last weeks of pregnancy, helps in natural childbirth. It is a calming herb and muscle relaxant.

BLESSED THISTLE (*Cnicus benedictus*)

Blessed thistle is a tonic for the female organs and a blood purifier to eradicate excess estrogen build-up. It balances hormones and can help with infertility. It will also help eliminate menopausal symptoms. Blessed thistle, along with red raspberry, helps increase mother's milk. It helps alleviate indigestion, which is common during pregnancy.

BLUE COHOSH (*Caulophyllum thalictriodes*)

This herb contains antispasmodic properties, helping relieve pain in menstrual cramps and childbirth. It is useful in cases of toxemia, in promoting menses, and in balancing estrogen. It is very useful in reducing emotional and nervous tension which is a very common women's problem.

Blue cohosh is one herb with a reputation of preventing miscarriage. It relaxes the uterus, eases pain and strengthens the uterus to prevent premature delivery. It is used in combinations, along with cramp bark, black cohosh, false unicorn, ginger, raspberry and blessed thistle.

BURDOCK (*Arctium lappa*)

Burdock is a great herb for cleansing the blood, and is very useful in cases of toxemia. It has mild diuretic properties to rid the kidneys of toxins. It increases sweat, urination and bile to clean the body. Burdock rids the liver of excess estrogen and helps to restore liver function. Its inulin content aids the pituitary gland in releasing an ample supply of protein to helps balance hormones.

CAT'S CLAW (*Uncaria tomentosa*)

Clinical research has found that cat's claw has the ability to reduce inflammation and work as an anti-inflammatory. It has also been use to help with gastrointestinal disorders such as gastritis, hemorrhoids, ulcers, parasites, Crohn's disease, and bowel problems, and has the ability to heal the entire digestive tract.

Cat's claw has the ability to act as an antioxidant in protecting the body from free radical damage and destroying or neutralizing carcinogens before they can damage the cells. It may inhibit the growth of cancer cells. It also is recognized in helping support the body during chemotherapy and radiation therapies for cancer. It has been used successfully to treat conditions associated with a weakened immune system such as AIDS, herpes, and Epstein Barr Syndrome.

Cat's claw can help protect cells from a number of potentially harmful environmental substances, including herbicides, pesticides, air pollution, X-ray treatments, rancid foods, alcohol, and stress.

CRAMP BARK (*Viburnum opulus*)

Cramp bark is used along with false unicorn and blue cohosh to help prevent miscarriage. It eases the pain of menstrual cramps and acts as a sedative and a tonic for the uterus. It is good for congestion and hardening of the liver. Cramp bark is a valuable herb to help prevent nervous disorders in pregnancy as well as "after-pain" of childbirth and cramps. It is useful for the cramping pains of pregnancy which occur in the legs and calves.

DONG QUAI (Angelica sinensis)

Dong quai is known and used extensively for its ability to help with female disorders. During pregnancy it is used to nourish the fetus with its rich supply of vitamins and minerals. It helps to dissolve blood clots and increases circulation. It has a tranquilizing effect on the central nervous system, nourishing the blood and brain.

Dong quai is truly a woman's herb, helping to increase energy and strengthen the entire body. It is used for all female complaints, including PMS, menopausal symptoms, cramps, backaches due to menstrual cramps and hot flashes. It improves digestion and assimilation, strengthens the nervous system, helps in stroke recovery and as a blood purifier, improves circulation, stimulates production of interferon, and boosts the immune system.

FALSE UNICORN (Chamailirum luteum)

This herb is used in herbal formulas to correct almost all problems of the female reproductive organs. It can help restore health and muscle tone to the uterus. It is used for menopausal problems and relieves headaches and depression. False unicorn helps to strengthen a weak stomach and improve digestion. It is used to treat infertility, both in men and women.

FEVERFEW (Chrysanthemum parthenium)

Feverfew is used to strengthen the uterus and help expel the afterbirth. It promotes menses, calms the nerves, and naturally relieves migraine headaches. It is excellent for relieving colds and inflammation of arthritis. It is used for dizziness, tinnitus and aids in circulation to the brain and head area.

HORSETAIL (*Equisetum arvense*)

Horsetail contains silicon, which converts to calcium in the body. Calcium is necessary for healthy nerve sheaths, veins and artery walls, bones, teeth, nails and hair. It helps to prevent osteoporosis and nourishes the kidneys and bladder.

Horsetail helps with internal bleeding, urinary and prostate disorders, bed-wetting, skin problems and lung disease. It is known to help dissolve tumors, strengthen the glands and aid in circulation.

LICORICE (*Glycyrrhiza glabra*)

Licorice is often used to treat a variety of female problems. Licorice stimulates the production of estrogen in the body, which is very useful during menopause. It helps normalize ovulation, strengthen the adrenal glands, and restore energy to the body. The properties in licorice help stimulate natural interferon in the body and strengthen the immune system. It contains both anti-inflammatory and anti-allergenic properties.

Licorice is used in hypoglycemia, diabetes, Addison's Disease, and lung problems. It also has the ability to help heal ulcers.

MILK THISTLE (*Silybum marianum*)

Milk thistle is an excellent liver cleanser, as well as a protector. Women are known to have more sluggish livers than men because they are prone to accumulate bad estrogen there. Milk thistle can be used with other herbs such as burdock to cleanse and boost liver health. Milk thistle contains flavonoids that have a strong liver protective action. The silymarin content counteracts a number of toxic substances including alcohol, acetaminophen, carbon tetrachloride and Amanita mushroom poison. Silymarin alters liver cell membranes and prevents toxins from passing through the cells.

Gerarde, a practicing herbalist in 1597, said that milk thistle was one of the best remedies for melancholy, to which depression and a sluggish liver are related.

RED CLOVER (*Trifolium pratense*)

Red clover is a great liver cleanser. When the liver is congested it has a negative effect on the nervous system and brain. It contains antibiotic properties, helping inhibit vaginal and breast infections. It is an excellent herb often used in formulas for cleansing the blood and cells. It has been used for treating cancer, bronchitis, nervous conditions, spasms and toxins in the body.

RED RASPBERRY (*Rubus idaeus*)

Red raspberry is famous for its benefits in female problems. One reason is that it is rich in iron. It is used in pregnancy to strengthen the uterus, prevent nausea and hemorrhage, reduce pain during childbirth and to enrich colostrum found in breast milk. It is an excellent herb to treat children for conditions such as colds, diarrhea, colic, fever and other childhood diseases.

Red raspberry also helps to nourish and strengthen all the glands and to prevent miscarriage. Red raspberry is rich in vitamins and minerals to nourish the mother and baby during pregnancy.

ST. JOHN'S WORT (*Hypericum perforatum*)

St. John's wort is a very effective treatment for depression and anxiety. It contains expectorant properties to eliminate toxins from the body, and helps keep the intestinal tract free from waste material.

It is also very effective for nervous system disorders such as traumas, neuralgia, sciatica, fibrositis, headaches, shingles, and back pain. It is useful for pains, insomnia, hysteria and depression after childbirth.

SARSAPARILLA (*Smilax ornata*)

Sarsaparilla contains properties to help the body produce progesterone and balance hormones. It helps in glandular balance to strengthen the entire body. Sarsaparilla is a blood purifier and is beneficial for skin conditions. It is used in formulas to strengthen the female organs.

VITEX (*Vitex agnus-castus*)

Vitex is considered a very beneficial herb for women's ailments. Scientific research has shown that the extract has the ability to help restore normal ovulation and menstrual cycles. It strengthens the pituitary to release hormones that balance estrogen and progesterone, mainly boosting the progesterone levels.

Vitex, like many other herbs, especially demonstrates its benefits after a few months' use. Its properties will strengthen the female organs. *Vitex* helps with water retention, emotional upsets, migraine headaches, mastitis, and menstrual cramps.

For fertility, it may be beneficial in regulating the ovulatory cycle. In menopause it can help with hot flashes, depression and dry vagina. The following herbal combination can help in women's problems: *Vitex*, wild yam, dong quai, dandelion, prickly ash, red raspberry, cramp bark and pau d'arco.

WILD YAM (*Dioscorea villosa*)

Wild yam is beneficial for balancing hormones. It stimulates the production of progesterone. It is a liver cleanser and is therefore useful for excess estrogen accumulation. Wild yam relaxes the muscles, soothes the nerves, and relieves pain in the uterine area. It helps in nausea and cramps, and aids in preventing miscarriage.

Wild yam contains diuretic properties to eliminate toxins from the kidneys. It helps cleanse the veins and prevent high blood pressure.

YELLOW DOCK (*Rumex crispus*)

A great woman's herb to help anemia, yellow dock can be used along with dandelion and kelp. It is rich in iron that the body can assimilate easily. It nourishes the spleen and liver and cleans the lymphatic system, which helps clean up skin eruptions.

Yellow dock is a beneficial herb for toxemia, infections, ulcers and wounds. It is considered one of the best blood builders in the herbal kingdom.

Toxic Shock Syndrome

Toxic Shock Syndrome primarily affects menstruating women in their late teens or early twenties. It afflicts those who use highly absorbent synthetic fiber tampons, which are associated with the proliferation of *Staphylococcus aureus*. This organism produces the toxins which cause the symptoms of toxic shock.

Many women have been stricken by this disease quite suddenly. In 1985, it was reported over the news that 114 women had died from this illness. These women usually experienced nausea, diarrhea and dizziness, accompanied by a sudden high fever. This was often followed by a rash, peeling skin, and possibly shock, unconsciousness, paralysis and even death. A sharp drop in blood pressure is another symptom of this syndrome. Recovery is often a long and painful process. Women who have had it can get it again and it is a possibility wherever staph organisms lurk.

In the book *The Home Health Advisor*, author Rita Elkins states:

> After certain types of tampons were taken off the market, toxic shock no longer received the kind of publicity we saw during the 80s. Today, several hundred cases are reported each year, although now, menstrual toxic shock comprises only a quarter of cases. The mortality rate from toxic shock is approximately 3 percent.

> The staphylococcus bacteria are believed to enter the body through a break in the skin and are sometimes present in the nose and mouth areas. Some women carry this bacteria within the vagina. The exact link of tampon use to the disease is unclear. One theory explaining the relationship of tampons to the infection is that they trap bacteria and provide a breeding ground in which they multiply rapidly.

> Leaving a tampon in for long periods of time affords the bacteria an opportunity to reproduce quickly. Another theory is that synthetic, absorbent fibers of some tampons can cause tiny lacerations in the vagina which allow for the transmission of the bacteria and the toxin it produces into the bloodstream. Toxic shock syndrome has also been associated with vaginal barrier contraceptives (diaphragms or

contraceptive sponges), and there have been some reports of sexual partners both contracting the disease. Toxic shock can occur as a result of staph infection of the skin, wounds, as a complication of surgery, influenza, pneumonia and from infections related to childbirth. Some cases of toxic shock syndrome have been linked to nasal packing and to control nosebleeds.

The November/December 1992 issue of the Canadian-based magazine, *Health Naturally*, featured an article entitled "Health Hazards of Tampons." It states:

Normally, the amount of toxin produced by the *Staphylococcus aureus* bacteria is not enough to cause a problem. Magnesium in the blood controls these toxic levels. Dr. Edward Kass of Harvard University, however, found that magnesium was severely depleted in all cases of TSS studied. As a result, the bacteria was able to produce toxin levels 20 times higher than normal.

It is not enough that women have to be concerned about the possibility of TSS and ulceration due to rayon fibers. There is added danger from dioxin created by chlorine bleaching...Chlorine bleaching creates dioxin, one of the most harmful, cancer-causing chemicals known.

Both the Department of the Environment in the UK and the U.S. Food and Drug Administration (FDA) claim that the amounts of dioxin found in tampons is well below currently acceptable levels. One U.S. senator on a congressional panel disagreed and accused the FDA of "ignoring the possible dangers to women from tampons that may contain dioxin, a toxic substance believed to cause cancer." The senator then stated emphatically, "No level of dioxin is acceptable!" . . . A woman during her lifetime will use approximately 10,000 tampons and/or pads. If we consider the small, so-called "acceptable levels" of dioxin in just one tampon and multiply by the number a woman will ultimately use, can anyone in clear conscience, really believe that dioxin at any level is acceptable?

Natural and Nutritional Treatments

The nervous system is connected to the immune system, and when one is weakened, the other becomes weak. Eat a nutritious diet and exercise often. Do not let stressful situations control how you act. Fresh, clean air is vital for the lungs and the entire immune system. Create happiness, love and peace within yourself.

A diet rich in vegetables such as broccoli, cabbage, cauliflower, brussels sprouts, parsley, green beans, corn, dark leaf lettuce, fresh peas, and sprouts; fruits such as apples, apricots, bananas, berries, cherries, melons, peaches, plums, and pineapple; and non-red meats such as chicken and fish are suggested.

Antioxidant nutrients can help fortify the body's immune system and strengthen cells and tissues. The following formula is an excellent example of antioxidant ingredients, especially combined to protect and sustain the immune system. It helps prevent toxins and poisons from invading the body and restores health diminished by the many diseases that plague us today. This formula contains bioflavonoids, grapefruit pectin, milk thistle extract, acerola fruit, and cruciferous vegetable concentrate.

Bioflavonoids work synergistically and enhance the absorption of vitamin C. They need to be replaced daily because the body cannot reproduce or store these nutrients. This formula has anti-inflammatory, anti-allergy and antiviral properties. It also helps the body produce its own interferon to fight off diseases.

Grapefruit Pectin is derived from the pulp and rind of the grapefruit. This pectin ingredient is one of the fibers that helps eliminate toxins from the body.

Milk Thistle Extract is a potent antioxidant that prevents free radical damage. It is very effective to protect the liver from the damage of cirrhosis or hepatitis. It will also help regenerate liver cells and restore normal liver function.

Acerola Fruit is derived from the acerola cherry, a tropical fruit which is very high in natural vitamin C. It enhances the activity of the bioflavonoids.

Cruciferous Vegetables contain very powerful phytonutrients that have been scientifically shown to balance hormones, detoxify the liver and intestinal tract, and reinforce the body's immune system.

Magnesium produces properdin, a blood protein that can help fight invading bacteria and viruses.

B-complex Vitamins protect the nervous system, prevent fatigue and increase resistance to disease.

Acidophilus is important if on antibiotic therapy for the replacement of friendly bacteria.

Chlorophyll helps to clear the blood of toxins.

Burdock helps to remove toxins from the bloodstream.

Cat's Claw contains powerful properties to help boost the body's ability to scavenge and destroy toxins and harmful bacteria.

Echinacea is a lymphatic and blood cleanser.

(*Note:* Nutritional and herbal suggestions are offered as supportive treatments. Toxic shock syndrome needs immediate medical treatment and requires the facilities of a hospital.)

Silicone Breast Implants

In the never-ending quest for beauty, vanity has its price — especially where silicone breast implants are concerned. Where nature hasn't provided, the surgeon promises to excel. From 1962 until 1988, (when press coverage began exposing the harm), silicone breast implants were hailed as the final answer to breast enlargement. Around 128,000 women were getting implants every year, and plastic surgeons were pocketing anywhere from $1,000 to $5,000 from each operation.

Now, disturbing evidence shows these implants are subject to rupture and leakage, and the escaping silicone can stimulate all kinds of harm within the body. The April 1996 issue of *Working Woman* reports: "Some physicians . . . report persistent, prevalent health problems among implanted women. 'When I have a patient with extreme pain in her right arm whose MRI shows silicone wrapped around a nerve,' says Dr. Steven Weiner, a Los Angeles rheumatologist on the

UCLA faculty, 'don't tell me the problems don't exist.' And Dr. Lu-Jean Feng, a Cleveland plastic surgeon who has performed more than 800 explantations (implant removals), reports a 68 percent rupture rate in implants more than 10 years old."

Jeffrey S. Bland, Ph.D., reports in the August, 1994 issue of *Let's Live* magazine: "In testing the blood of women with silicone breast implants, Randall M. Goldblum, M.D., professor of pediatrics and human biological chemistry at the University of Texas Medical Center, has detected antibodies that respond to particulate silicone, which has been released into the bloodstream (*The Lancet,* Aug. 29, 1992; 340:510). In another test, about half of a group of women with silicone breast implants had greatly elevated antibody levels to silicone in their bloodstream levels, which may be associated with inflammation and autoimmune diseases (Plastic Surgery Forum, 1990; vol. 8:13).

The body will distribute this substance via the bloodstream into the tissues of the joints, muscles and brain. The body will react against this foreign invader and the result may be chronic fatigue syndrome, and autoimmune disorder symptoms such as those associated with lupus or multiple sclerosis. According to Carolyn DeMarco, M.D., as quoted in *Health Naturally* (August/September 1996 issue): "Other symptoms include memory loss, poor concentration, sleep disorders, severe weight loss, hair loss, liver dysfunction, lymph node swelling, weakness, breast and nipple inflammation, circulation problems, joint pains, chronic muscle pain and stiffness."

Dr. DeMarco goes on to explain:

> Before healing can begin, the transplant first has to be removed. Secondly, a detoxification program must be started including supervised modified fasting, colon therapy, baths with ozonated water, and lymphatic massage. Other aspects of treatment include antioxidant supplements, cellulase enzymes, nutrients to support the liver and kidneys, and intravenous vitamin and mineral therapy.

> This, at least, is the successful program developed by Dr. Lee Cowden in Dallas, Texas. Treatment should always be supervised by a qualified practitioner. Dr. Cowden says in *Alternative Medicine Digest* that 'Women going through this detoxification program process see white powdery flakes coming out of their urine and stools

. . . after which their symptoms start to lift and dramatically improve. Finally, I personally believe it is much more important to work on befriending our bodies than to cater to socially defined images of how women's bodies should look."

Estrogen

The body depends on substances known as steroid hormones for many functions. They are produced in tiny amounts and are used in specific areas of the body. Estrogens are members of this larger family, and the main estrogen is known as estradiol. This is the substance that is usually referred to as "estrogen."

Estrogen is produced mainly by the ovaries and is responsible for many changes in the female body, including determining the time of the onset of puberty. Estrogens are formed in the ovaries, mainly from the androgen precursor hormone, testosterone. Estrogen causes the growth of mammary (breast) tissues and the deposition of fat in the breasts. It also regulates the deposit of fat in other areas of the body such as buttocks and thighs. Estrogens keep the skin soft and smooth, unlike the "male" steroid hormones (androgens) which cause it to become tough and thick. Estrogen does this by encouraging the formation of collagen, the protein support structure underlying the skin. Estrogen can also stimulate bone growth, and this is why many women experience a "growth spurt" at puberty. Estrogen also causes the bones of the pelvis to flatten and widen, giving them the graceful curves representative of entry into womanhood.

In the book *How to Reduce Your Risk of Breast Cancer*, Dr. Jon J. Michnovicz explains how estrogen works in the body:

The production, activity, breakdown, and elimination of estrogen in a woman's body may be conceptualized as four steps of a single biological pathway. We call this the "estrogen pathway." The steps of the "estrogen pathway" can be outlined as follows:

1. Estrogen is produced in the body.
2. Estrogen circulates throughout the body.

3. Estrogen binds to the estrogen receptor.
4. Estrogen is broken down and eliminated.

Estrogen binds to the estrogen receptor in breast cells. This is an extremely important process by which estrogen is "captured" from the bloodstream by a specialized cell protein able to recognize only estrogen. The estrogen receptors are present within cells of several tissues of a woman's body. Most are found in the breasts and the uterus, with lesser amounts in the skin, bone, brain, and liver.

Once an active estrogen molecule binds to the estrogen receptor, that cell's DNA becomes activated. As a result, the cell may grow. This process can be compared to a car engine's lock and key: An estrogen hormone acts like the key; the estrogen receptor is the lock and the cell's DNA is like the engine. Once the key (estrogen) is inserted, the lock (receptor) is opened and the engine turns on (DNA is activated).

Once the body has used the estrogen it needs, the excess is broken down and excreted from the body via the urine and intestines (although small amounts are retained in the intestines and recycled through the body to continue helping it with its estrogen needs).

Dr. Michnovicz explains that research shows there are two major by-products of estrogen breakdown called the C-16 metabolite and the C-2 metabolite. C-2 is inactivated by the body, while C-16 remains very potent and can attack the DNA of breast cells and cause breast cancer. Further studies show that there are substances in fruits and vegetables called phytochemicals that can reduce the body's formation of the harmful C-16 estrogen and increase its production of the harmless C-2 form of the hormone. (Elsewhere in this book, for simplification, we have referred to C-16 as the "bad" estrogen.) Dr. Michnovicz goes on to say:

There is an important link between the dietary fiber a woman eats and the estrogen in her body. After estrogen hormones have done their necessary work in the breasts and other cells, they must be properly eliminated. If not, estrogen would continue to accumulate in the body and might eventually reach dangerously high levels. It is the function of the intestines and the kidneys to dispose of excessive estrogen.

Women are often surprised to learn they normally excrete a large percentage of the body's estrogen each day in their bowel movements. These intestinal estrogens are sent from the liver into the intestines as part of the bile and then eliminated. However, the contents of the intestines may take up to twenty-four hours (or more) to pass through the body. There is plenty of time, therefore, for a significant proportion of the intestinal estrogen to be reabsorbed back into the body. This reabsorption of estrogen from the intestines is greatly affected by the amount of fiber you eat each day.

THE ESTROGEN CONNECTION TO CANCER OF THE BREASTS, OVARIES AND UTERUS

Diet plays an integral part in the development of cancer. Sugar turns to fat in the body and high fat consumption has been linked to breast cancer. Toxins are stored in animal fats and women who consume a lot of dairy products and meats, and eat very little fiber and vegetables are at the highest risk, just by virtue of their dietary habits. Since fat is a repository for toxins, and a woman's breast is comprised mostly of fatty tissue, toxins — including "bad" estrogen — can accumulate there until the time bomb detonates. The old adage, "An ounce of prevention is worth a pound of cure," certainly applies in this case.

There is alarming evidence that chemicals that can mimic estrogen in the body, also creating havoc and harm. In the March 1996 issue of *Let's Live* magazine, Betty Franklin reports: "Xenoestrogens is the term coined by distinguished and maverick epidemiologist, Devra Lee Davis. She has argued for over 15 years that man-made chemicals can act like hormones in the body, mimicking estrogen, or blocking the male hormone, testosterone. And evidently, according to the ultimate hormone authority, in my view, John R. Lee, M.D., all-important progesterone production is affected, which is bad news, because this biologically counters excessive estrogen. Petrochemicals — specifically insecticides — are the culprits, contaminating environments in all industrialized countries, and increasing cancers, along with affecting our hormones."

Health author Amanda Spake is quoted in the October 1995 issue of *Health* magazine, also speaking of Devra Lee Davis:

Davis believes that a vast number of man-made chemicals — in some pesticides used on crops and lawns, and in some cosmetics and plastic bottles, among other things — can behave in the body like hormones, mimicking estrogen or blocking testosterone.

For decades, animal biologists have been drawing similar conclusions, documenting the fact that pollutants can destroy animals' ability to reproduce and can reduce their immunity to disease. Once considered outlandish, that evidence is no longer debated. Scientists believe that one of the forms of estrogen women make naturally — estradiol — activates estrogen receptors, stimulating breast cell growth and, sometimes, damaging cell DNA. If a woman begins menstruating early, enters menopause late, never gets pregnant, never breast-feeds, or is obese, she'll be exposed to more estradiol, increasing her risk of breast cancer.

"We used to believe that only a woman's natural estrogen could turn the key on these receptors and cause breast cancer," Davis says . . . "It is now clear that many chemicals in plastics and pesticides can turn the key as well."

Another scary aspect related to estrogen and the environment is described in the December 1994/January 1995 issue of *Health Naturally*. David Suzuki, Ph.D., says,

During the 1970s when "the pill" had become a major form of contraception, I half jokingly asked a physiologist how much synthetic estrogen could end up in the sewers. Doing a very rough calculation, he estimated an annual output of tons in Canada alone. I suggested in jest there might not be a population problem in the future.

But what seemed like science fiction may now be science fact. British media reports about estrogen pollution in drinking water have triggered near panic among residents living along London's River Thames. Hermaphroditic fish are being caught in the Thames, sometimes reaching 40 percent of the catches where urban sewage flows in. A higher incidence of male sterility in humans has also been noted. Some three million women who live near the river regularly take "the pill." That means up to 800 million pills a year could ultimately pass into the river and end up in the drinking water.

During menopause the adrenal glands can take over with estrogen production, if they are healthy. Dr. Jon R. Michnovicz explains in the book, *How to Reduce Your Risk of Breast Cancer:* "As endocrinologists learned to measure the minute levels of hormones in the body, they discovered that estrogen is still present in older women, though at very low levels. In post-menopausal women, the adrenal glands become of the source of large quantities of estrogen building blocks, converted in fat cells to active estrogen."

Endometriosis

Endometriosis is a rather common disease in our present era. It is estimated that 40 to 50 percent of women who undergo hysterectomies have endometriosis. It is an outgrowth of the uterine lining into the pelvic cavity, which can cause irregular bleeding, pain during intercourse and menses, severe pelvic pain and even infertility.

This condition was discovered in 1899 and described in medical journals. In 1920, Dr. J.A. Sampson described the ever increasing disease as very serious. Dr. Sampson found clumps of brown, sticky tissue and old, clotted blood adhering in unusual places: ovaries, rectal ligaments, intestines and fallopian tubes. In severe cases, the abdominal organs were glued together and twisted out of place by the contortions of the unusual and strange tissue. Then he discovered that the sticky clotted tissue was the same as that which lined the normal uterus. It also reacted to the hormonal cycle the same way as the uterine tissue, proliferating when stimulated by estrogen, and actually bleeding during menstruation.

The reason it is hard to diagnose is that it can appear and disappear according to the hormonal profile of the woman. It is not fully understood how the tissue escapes from the uterus in the first place.

We believe that the reason we are seeing more of this disease is because of the excess estrogen we are getting in beef, chicken, turkeys and in all dairy products: milk, butter, cottage cheese, cream cheese, sour cream and whipping cream. We feel that the body would be able to handle excess toxins such as artificial hormones if the colon were kept healthy and regular. What happens is the liver becomes over-loaded because the bowels are clogged and backed up with wastes. Toxins enter the bloodstream, causing problems in the estrogen-receptor areas; namely, the breasts, uterus, vagina and other related parts. *Candida albicans* yeast infection is another culprit. It can produce poisons in the body and confuse hormone messages, creating a hormone imbalance.

In 1984, an epidemic of early puberty was reported in both males and females all across Puerto Rico. United States health authorities also reported enlarged breasts in pre-teen children in parts of the continental United States. Dr. Saenz de Rodriguez in Puerto Rico had seen many cases of premature puberty for several years. She became convinced that the children were being contaminated with estrogen, where four and five-year-old girls were suffering from enlarged breasts and ovarian cysts. Milk products, beef and poultry were found to be the problem. The doctor said, "We are supposed 'to mind our manners' and not question the effects that drugs have upon the population, or your colleagues call you a troublemaker." She went on to say, "Much of what we consider healthful growth in our youngsters could be similar to the fattening process the ranchers now use for their cattle. We should not, however, underestimate the time-bomb that is present in those skyrocketing sales figures for fried chicken and hamburgers among young people."

DIETARY GUIDELINES AND NATURAL TREATMENT

A good diet can help detoxify excessive estrogen. Take blood purification and lower bowel therapy herbal formulas. They will clean and purify the body of excess estrogen and other toxins. Change to a diet using fresh juices from vegetables and fruits.

Steamed and fresh vegetables are delicious. Use fresh salads made from leaf lettuce, cabbage, carrots, broccoli and other vegetables. Use olive oil and lemon juice for dressing, with added garlic, onions, parsley, and vegetable seasoning. Use brown rice, millet, buckwheat, and all whole grains (thermos cooking will retain the enzymes and B-complex vitamins). Exercise is very beneficial to prevent adhesions from adhering to the walls of the uterus and other organs. It also helps to normalize hormone levels by metabolizing fat.

NUTRITIONAL SUPPLEMENTS

Vitex agnus-castus can promote hormone balance in a woman's body.

Cat's Claw can help detoxify the intestinal tract.

Dong Quai has been named the "queen" of all female herbs. It nourishes the female glands and helps to strengthen all internal body organs and systems.

Essential Fatty Acids can help balance glandular function throughout the body.

Black Cohosh provides natural "phyto" or plant estrogen-like substances.

Wild Yam helps balance the glands and promote hormone harmony in the body. Wild yam cream is not an internal supplement, but it has demonstrated remarkable abilities to balance levels of hormones in the body by applying it externally. It provides a natural source of progesterone which works with estrogen to create a synergistic team to alleviate symptoms of PMS and menopause and even help with osteoporosis.

Saw Palmetto can regulate the menstrual cycle and relieve painful periods.

Dandelion benefits liver function and stimulates it to detoxify poisons.

Cruciferous Vegetable Concentrate is a supplement ingredient that helps balance hormones and detoxify the bad estrogen in the liver and intestinal tract.

"Good" and "Bad" Fats

Fats are important for health! Also known as "lipids", they help balance the body's chemistry and provide padding as protection for vital organs. Fats provide a source of energy for body processes and they help with the transportation and absorption of fat-soluble vitamins such as A, D, E, and K. They are also a source of the vital nutrients known as essential fatty acids.

Women need to understand the importance of the body's requirement for specific fats and oil in their diet. There are some fats that are essential for hormone balance. There are those that interfere with the body's ability to excrete excess estrogen, and interfere with the production of essential hormones.

Eating a high-fat diet stimulates the over production of hormones, especially "bad" estrogen that harms the breast, ovaries and uterus. The bad fats prevent the essential fatty acids from protecting the cells. Trans-fatty acids are toxic substances that are formed when oils are refined (many oils on the market shelves are refined). When oils are heated, it changes their structure so they do not nourish the cells, but collect in the arteries, and other parts of the body.

Bad fats prevent natural fats from entering the cells and create free radical damage. Trans-fatty acids are sticky. They cause clumping of the blood cells and block enzymes from producing prostaglandins. Bad fats reduce oxygen supply to the cells. They also destroy the myelin sheath protecting the nervous system.

The bad fats are found in all processed foods. Even whole wheat products become rancid when exposed to air. When the labels on food contain "hydrogenated," in any form, it is the bad oil.

Packaged mixes, potato chips, cookies, cakes, french fries, breads, pies, rolls, pastries, crackers, candy, and frosting mixes are just a few of the products that contain bad fats. There is no way to tell how long the packaged food has been on the shelves. Even fresh bakery goods can be made from trans-fatty acids and rancid grains. Chocolate is high in fat, and is made worse because of the high amount of sugar needed to make it palatable. Bad fats include lard, margarine, vegetable oil, (that have been heated), and shortening.

Some people shy away from anything that has the word "fatty" associated with it because they think it will make them gain unnecessary weight. However, there are "good fats" that can actually help decrease the desire to eat the harmful ones.

Fats are solid at room temperature, and oils are those which are liquid at room temperature. Stay away from fats in which the normal, health-giving properties have been altered to the point where they actually cause damage to the body's cells. Even natural elements such as light, oxygen and heat can cause the breakdown and rancidity of fats. The composition of extremely heated fats, especially those of vegetable origin, will turn into cancer-causing agents by causing free-radical damage to the body. Ideally, a health-minded person will not eat deep-fried foods, as these are especially dangerous. However, because we are all human and it is almost impossible to eat a perfect diet in today's world, taking essential fatty acid supplements will help offset the damage done to the body by the "bad fats."

ESSENTIAL FATTY ACIDS

Essential fatty acids are vital nutritional components that our bodies need for many functions. They are found in the seeds of plants and in the oils of cold-water fish. Essential fatty acids, sometimes referred to as vitamin F, cannot be made by the body — they must be supplied in the diet. Many factors, including stress, allergies, disease, and a diet high in fried foods can increase the body's nutritional need for essential fatty acids.

Essential fatty acids make up the outer membrane of every cell in our bodies. Here they strengthen and fortify these tissues against the invasion of viruses, bacteria and allergy-causing substances. The health of the cell membrane depends upon adequate amounts of EFAs. The benefits of essential fatty acids on human health include:

- reducing serum cholesterol levels
- lowering triglyceride levels
- helping to clear away existing plaque from arterial walls
- preventing abnormal blood clotting by inhibiting the production of a substance known as thromboxane, which allows platelets to clot
- lowering blood pressure
- altering the production of leukotrienes which aggravate inflammation in the body. This has shown to beneficial, especially to those suffering from conditions such as arthritis, lupus, psoriasis and other related ailments
- the ability to help with many chronic, stubborn conditions, such as alcoholism, breast cancer, cardiovascular disease, premenstrual syn-

drome, rheumatoid arthritis, and assisting in the proper management of weight

Essential fatty acids are found in both plant and animal sources. The oils of cold water fish such as salmon, bluefish, herring, tuna, mackerel and similar fish are known as Omega-3 fatty acids. The fresh-pressed oils of many raw seeds and nuts (such as black currant, borage, flax and evening primrose) contain Omega-6 fatty acids. Processing destroys the nourishing aspects of essential fatty acids and creates what are known as "trans-fatty acids."

DANGERS OF FRIED FOODS

You would think that liquid oils are healthier for you than solid fats. Well, this is not true when it comes to frying. Because saturated fats are more stable than unsaturated fats when it comes to exposure to light, heat and air, they are more desirable than oils for frying. However, the ideal way to prepare food for frying is to do it like the Chinese do, by stir frying. The Chinese put water into the pan or wok and then the oil, then the vegetables and meat, constantly stirring the mixture around the entire time. This keeps the temperature of the oil lower. It also protects it from oxidation by forming steam which helps keep air from degenerating the oil.

In many commercial restaurants and fast-food establishments, oil is repeatedly re-used at high temperatures. It soon becomes dark and rancid, exhibiting a strong odor and flavor. Many toxic substances can form when oils are heated to high temperatures. One of these is "trans-fatty acids." These substances are deformed fat molecules which can damage the cells and cause a fatty acid deficiency by inhibiting enzymes that cause fatty acids to be changed into essential molecules. This may, in turn, interfere with prostaglandin production and cause problems with blood pressure and normal platelet action. The body cannot use trans-fatty acids for utilization so they just collect around fatty tissues and the body's organs. They also take up space where essential fatty acids normally would be, but do not perform any useful function. It is best to avoid frying food; if needed, use the Chinese method, or use a small amount of saturated fat (such as olive oil or butter) heated only to a moderately high temperature.

Cholesterol — A Good Thing

The much-maligned body substance known as cholesterol has received a bad rap in the press. Cholesterol, a "waxy alcohol," is actually necessary for many vital bodily functions. It is found in the bile, blood, brain tissue, liver, kidneys, adrenal glands, and myelin sheaths (insulating material) of nerve fibers. It helps the body absorb and transport fatty acids and is necessary for the body to synthesize vitamin D. It is also a building material for hormones produced by the adrenal and reproductive glands. The body will actually manufacture its own cholesterol to ensure a continuous supply of this important fat. In the book *The Complete Book of Fats and Oils,* author Lewis Harrison explains:

> There are many essential vitamins, hormones, and chemical compounds that are derived from cholesterol or that require cholesterol for their manufacture. Three hormones that are manufactured from cholesterol are steroid (or sex) hormones, aldosterone, and cortisone.

> Of the steroid hormones produced from cholesterol, the best known are estrogen and progesterone in women and testosterone in men. During pregnancy the placenta will manufacture cholesterol. The cholesterol is needed to produce progesterone, which keeps the pregnancy from terminating. Estrogen, progesterone, and testosterone are essential to the development and maintenance of the physical attributes associated with each sex.

The "fight or flight" hormone called cortisone is produced from cholesterol. Cortisone helps the body's defense system by acting as an anti-inflammatory agent. The body synthesizes cholesterol throughout the body. It is manufactured by cells, glands, small intestines and the liver. Cholesterol is constructed from dietary by products of proteins, sugars and fats. If the diet contains excessive fats, especially the saturated types, the body will convert it into cholesterol. People who eat highsugar or -fat diets may experience elevated cholesterol levels.

Menopause

Menopause is the physical and emotional transition that marks the permanent cessation of menstruation. It usually begins between the ages of forty-five and fifty, and lasts approximately five years. It can take longer if a woman is in poor mental and physical health. However, if a woman is in good health, has properly functioning digestive and eliminative systems and a positive mental attitude, these symptoms are greatly minimized.

SYMPTOMS

- hot flashes
- night sweats
- depression
- dizziness
- headaches
- difficult breathing
- heart palpitations
- irritability
- mental confusion
- vaginal dryness

CAUSES

Some women start menopause early, and others later. Menopause is a normal transition in life. However, some fertility pills, contraceptives, and strong drugs can throw women into menopause long before its time, as can complete hysterectomies. Diminished hormone production has been associated with diseases in the post-menopausal years. They include heart disease and brittle bones (osteoporosis).

NATURAL TREATMENT

Following menopause, the ovaries continue to produce a reduced amount of estrogen. But with good nutrition, other glands can take over, such as the adrenals. If they are healthy, they begin to form a type of female hormone that complements the diminished amount of ovarian estrogen. There are so many side-effects from using estrogen replacement therapy that it is wise to investigate the natural route for many reasons. The side-effects from taking conjugated estrogen tablets include:

- nausea, vomiting; pain, cramps, swelling, or tenderness in the abdomen
- yellowing of the skin or whites of the eyes
- breast tenderness or enlargement
- enlargement of benign tumors of the uterus
- breakthrough bleeding or spotting
- change in amount of cervical secretion
- vaginal yeast infections
- retention of excess fluid (which may make some conditions worsen, such as asthma, epilepsy, migraine, heart disease or kidney disease)
- a spotty darkening of the skin, particularly on the face; reddening of the skin; skin rashes
- headache, migraines, dizziness, faintness, or changes in vision (including intolerance to contact lenses)
- mental depression
- involuntary muscle spasms
- hair loss or abnormal hairiness
- increase or decrease in weight
- changes in sex drive
- possible changes in blood sugar

Certain dietary foods and herbs can help the body continue producing the correct amount of necessary hormones, even progesterone. See "Nutritional Supplements" in this sub-section.

DIETARY GUIDELINES

Less calories are needed at this time of life. If they aren't decreased, there is a strong chance that excessive weight gain may result. If complex carbohydrates are added to the diet, with lots of vegetables and green salads plus increased exercise, the body can compensate for the weight gain. Soybeans and products can help reduce menopausal symptoms. The British medical journal *Lancet* (May 16, 1992; 339:1233) reported that plant estrogens (phytoestrogens) from soy in the diets of Japanese women may help to explain why they have minimized menopausal symptoms as compared to women who live in North America. Author Peter Jaret reports in the October, 1995 issue of *Health* magazine:

> . . . there's evidence that an estrogen-like substance (or phytoestrogen) found in soybeans can relieve some side effects of menopause and even slow down osteoporosis. What's more, it might cut the risk of many forms of cancer. "Wouldn't that be wonderful?" says Kesler, a trim woman in her mid-fifties who lives on a farm north of town. Like others she has fretfully watched her cholesterol climb since menopause, and she's concerned about osteoporosis. Still, she's reluctant to go on estrogen therapy. "My mother died of breast cancer," she says, "and it worries me that estrogen might raise my risk." By comparing before-and-after bone scans, [researchers] will also investigate whether soy foods can really retard osteoporosis as scientists suspect. Based on animal studies, the premise hinges on those estrogen look-alikes in soy. Called isoflavones, these bear so strong a resemblance to the hormone in a woman's body that they may be able to fill in when her own levels start to fall . . . several as-yet-unpublished studies suggest that isoflavones can alleviate hot flashes and night sweats in menopausal women, according to Mark Messina, a former program director in the Diet and Cancer branch of the National Cancer Institute who recently organized the first international symposium on soy foods and health. While more studies are needed, he's optimistic: "I'd bet good money soy protein will become a widely accepted alternative to estrogen replacement therapy within the next few years." [For more information, see subsection on "Estrogen."]

NUTRITIONAL SUPPLEMENTS

Black Cohosh is used as a tonic for the central nervous system. It helps in hot flashes and stimulates the secretions of the liver, kidneys and lymphatic system.

Blessed Thistle helps balance the hormones and is useful for headaches associated with menopause.

Damiana helps with hot flashes, hormone imbalance and diminished sex drive.

Dong Quai helps balance hormones and nourishes the female glands. It also helps alleviate nervousness, headaches and hot flashes.

Suma contains two plant hormones, sitosterol and stipmasterol, found beneficial in human metabolism by increasing heart circulation and decreasing high cholesterol levels in the blood. Sitosterol enhances the body's natural production of estrogen when the body is depleted.

Wild Yam is a hormone balancer and contains a natural source of progesterone.

False Unicorn is important for menopausal problems because of its effect in uterine disorders, headaches and depression.

Calcium, Magnesium, Silica and Boron are minerals which will help build strong bones and will enhance the body's utilization and absorption of plant estrogens to prevent osteoporosis. Boron is a trace mineral recently spotlighted by scientists who have found that it may be helpful in the preventing post-menopausal osteoporosis. Mostly found in plant foods, boron's nutritional effects in humans are becoming increasingly recognized and appreciated.

In a recent study, twelve post-menopausal women between the ages of forty-eight and eighty-two were closely monitored by researchers for twenty-four weeks. During the first seventeen weeks, the women consumed a low-boron diet. The following seven weeks, their diet was augmented with 3 milligrams daily of boron in the form of sodium borate capsules.

In a little over a week after receiving boron supplementation, the women dramatically decreased their body's excretion of both calcium and magnesium. They also experienced a substantial increase — about twice — the production of an active form of estrogen and testosterone. This indicates that boron supplementation can prevent calcium loss and bone demineralization in post-menopausal women. Additional follow-up research is currently in progress (Gaby, Alan R. *Preventing and Reversing Osteoporosis.* Prima, 1994).

FACTS AT A GLANCE

- Menopause usually begins between the ages of forty-five and fifty.
- Certain dietary foods and herbs can help the body continue producing the correct amount of necessary hormones.
- Soybeans and soy products can help reduce menopausal symptoms.
- Natural plant estrogens are called "phyto-estrogens."

Pregnancy

Pregnancy can be a very happy experience if the mother's body is free from toxins. Toxins can cause nausea and hormonal imbalances. Toxemia is common and a very dangerous condition for both the mother and the baby. Hormonal imbalances are due to constipation, with the liver failing to eliminate toxins faster than they accumulate. Even before becoming pregnant, parents should learn more about their bodies and the importance of a healthy diet and the dangers of drugs, caffeine and alcohol. Even over-the-counter drugs like aspirin seem harmless, but can cause birth defects in the early months of pregnancy. Women on diets high in junk foods have a greater incidence of difficult labors, premature babies, birth defects, infections, hemorrhages, nursing problems, and general problems during pregnancy.

There are many complaints of pregnancy which can be remedied naturally without resorting to drugs or over-the-counter remedies. Constipation, morning sickness, leg cramps, indigestion, fatigue, swollen ankles, varicose veins and backache are a few of the problems that pregnant women encounter that can be taken care of naturally.

Natural Treatment

Pregnancy is a normal function for a woman. It is essential to adopt a natural diet to provide nutrients for mother and baby alike. A good healthy body doesn't just happen; you have to work at it. Learn the importance of food in obtaining vitamins, minerals and nutrients that assist in the development of a healthy fetus. Blood purification is essential; using herbs and green drinks will help nourish the mother and baby. Exercise will help supply oxygen for the fetus as well as strengthen the mother for easier birth.

Dietary Guidelines

Protein is essential, and grains such as buckwheat and millet are complete proteins. Oats, yellow corn meal, barley and all grains are good.

A high-fiber diet will keep the bowels functioning properly, as well as supply nutrients needed for mother and baby. Grains, nuts and seeds contain properties that help increase immunity to disease. Acidophilus and natural yogurt will help provide good bacteria to prevent vaginal infections and constipation. Seeds are high in calcium and other minerals; flax, sesame; chia and pumpkin are the best. Fresh, steamed or baked vegetables such as potatoes, yams, squash and green beans are important. Raw vegetable or fruit salads add nutrition and variety. Some women experience infections after delivery of the baby, including mastitis (breast infection) while nursing. A folk remedy — if you feel mastitis coming on (painful, hot, firm and sore areas in the breast) — is to take a glass of water and add two to three tablespoons of apple cider vinegar with three tablespoons of honey. Stir well, keep refrigerated and sip during the day. (It will be strong-tasting and you may want to adjust the dosage of the vinegar a little). This remedy has helped stop mastitis in its tracks for some nursing mothers.

Alcohol passes freely through the placenta and is very toxic to the fetus. Chemicals such as preservatives, additives, food coloring, pesticides, monosodium glutamate and aspartame sweetener should be avoided. Drugs overwork the liver. Aspirin interferes with the clotting of blood. Antibiotics hinder the production of RNA and protein and could cause damage to the fetus. Drugs can also cause jaundice, respiratory difficulties, deformed limbs, mental retardation, and digestive problems. Smoking is very harmful. The carbon monoxide prevents the intake of oxygen in the fetus and could cause birth defects and premature births. It can cause stunted growth, low birth weight and hyperactive children. Avoid sugar, white flour products and fried foods. They rob the body of nutrients.

Nutritional Supplements

Vitamin A promotes growth and protects against toxins.

B-complex Vitamins protect the body from exhaustion and irritability, and strengthen the brain and heart. Extra B-6 controls swelling and nausea. B-12 creates more energy.

Vitamin C helps enhance contractions and minimize stretch marks. It protects the embryo from virus particles in the mother's tissues.

Vitamin D is essential to help calcium absorb. It is vital for bone and tooth development and helps develop jaw bones so the teeth have room for proper growth.

Vitamin E reduces the body's need for oxygen and strengthens the circulatory system. It helps prevent miscarriage.

Minerals are essential. If even one mineral is lacking, it could cause birth defects. Calcium is required more during pregnancy and a deficiency is caused by a high-meat diet.

Iron builds the blood and is important for the health of the baby's liver.

Yellow Dock contains forty percent easily assimilated iron.

Silicon and Magnesium help the body utilize calcium.

Selenium, Potassium and Zinc nourish the immune system.

Alfalfa contains protein, vitamins and minerals. It is also a blood cleanser. It is high in vitamin K, which clots the blood and prevents hemorrhaging.

Red Raspberry Leaf tea is high in iron and calcium and helps prepare the uterine muscles for delivery, especially if taken the last three months of pregnancy. However, it can help alleviate morning sickness during the first trimester.

Mint Teas will also help nausea.

Dandelion and Kelp are high in essential vitamins and minerals. Dandelion cleans and protects the liver. Kelp cleans the veins and provides nourishment.

The following herbs can be taken in combination during the last six weeks of pregnancy to facilitate a safe and easier delivery: black cohosh, red raspberry, squaw vine, blessed thistle, pennyroyal and lobelia.

FACTS AT A GLANCE

- A healthy pregnancy can be achieved through regular exercise.
- A nutritious diet is essential for a healthy pregnancy.
- Nourishing supplements can greatly benefit a pregnancy.
- Avoiding drugs, alcohol, smoking and junk foods will greatly reduce risks of early delivery and birth defects in the baby.

Fertility

After a girl reaches puberty, now around 11 or 12 (it used to be around 16 about 50 years ago), one egg is released each month until menopause. If the egg is not fertilized by male sperm, the egg is eliminated out of the body and a new one is released the next month. With infertility it is obvious that something has gone wrong to either the female egg or the male sperm.

Since infertility is increasing in occurrence, many couples experience unhappiness and frustration. It is now known that it is not necessarily the woman's fault, as was thought in the past. To be barren was a disgrace, and a woman was not considered a complete person. Not so today; men are to blame in about 40 percent of infertility cases.

CAUSES

Infertility in women can be caused by infections, venereal disease, inherited disorders, mishandled abortions, bacterial organisms, endometriosis, drugs, plugged fallopian tubes or nutritional deficiencies. And there are many more reasons. Birth control pills have been linked to permanent infertility, as well as high blood pressure, blood clots, strokes, heart disease, kidney failure, varicose veins, and cancer of the breast, uterus and liver. Infertility in men can be caused by overheating of the testes by hot temperatures (as in hot baths) and tight underpants. Sperm production can be affected by infections, hormone imbalance, being overweight and underweight, and exposure to toxins, such as smoking, drugs, alcohol, chemicals, stress and radiation (such as from X-rays). Also, the woman may have an overactive thyroid, causing an elevated body temperature, thus creating a less than optimal environment for the sperm.

NATURAL TREATMENT

Suggested herbal combinations include blood purifier, bone, anti-yeast (*Candida*), digestive, female glandular, immune system, lower bowels and nervine formulas. Autointoxication could be a problem. Change the diet to natural, wholesome foods. Sprouts and seeds, as well as nuts, fresh salads (using lots of green-leaf lettuce), cabbage and other raw vegetables have life-giving properties. Wheatgrass juice is an excellent food to build and clean the blood. Avoid chlorinated water, chemicals, pesticides, and herbicides. Avoid heavy metal poisoning. Check for mercury and other metal poisoning in the teeth. Stress has been implicated as a possible deterrent to conceiving. Try to slow down and take time out to relax. Stress triggers the fight or flight response through the pituitary, which also regulates the ovaries via the pituitary gland. Some women don't ovulate when under a lot of stress. Make sure that intercourse occurs during your "fertile" period, which is anywhere from 10 to 14 days from the start of your last period, if you are on a 28-day cycle. You will notice an increased mucus discharge during this "fertile" time. (For more information, read *Overcoming Infertility Naturally*, by Karen Bradstreet. This book describes in additional detail the relationship between nutrition, emotions and reproduction.)

DIETARY GUIDELINES

Eat fresh raw fruit first thing in the morning. The juice of one-half lemon in warm water is a liver booster. Soak whole grains the night before and eat for breakfast. Make almond milk for the cereal. Carrot and beet juices are nourishing. Raw and steamed vegetables, as well as the sprouts of alfalfa, mung beans, wheat, fenugreek, and radish are excellent. Organic fish, chicken and eggs are also nutritious.

NUTRITIONAL SUPPLEMENTS

Vitamin A assists in maintaining normal glandular activity and prevents sterility.

B-complex Vitamins protect against toxemia. They stabilize female hormone levels, which is critical in conceiving.

Vitamin C with bioflavonoids strengthen male sperm and female eggs. They protect against germs and viruses. Lack of this nutrient can cause varicose veins, slow healing of wounds and frequent sickness.

Vitamin E is called the fertility vitamin for the male as well as the female. Lack of vitamin E is the major cause of premature babies. It helps to prevent miscarriage. Dr. Evan Shute, famous doctor and researcher, found in years of treating his obstetrical patients that when he gave vitamin E to those who were pregnant and had a history of spontaneous abortion, they carried the fetus full-term and had healthy, normal babies. Dr. Shute said that vitamin E is vital because it is involved in the cardiovascular attachment of the developing fetus to the womb wall. Vitamin E has also been recommended for the husband, as well as the wife, to improve the quality of a man's sperm, which is essential to conception.

Selenium, Silicon, Calcium, Magnesium, Manganese and Zinc are critical for conceiving.

Damiana and Red Raspberry strengthen reproductive organs.

Dong Quai nourishes female reproductive system.

False Unicorn helps promote fertility.

Sarsaparilla stimulates the body's production of progesterone.

The following accounts are two cases in which women gave up fertility pills in favor of vitamin E, herbs and vitamins. Ann had tried for four years to become pregnant without success. She had seen two medical doctors who specialize in fertility. She took all kinds of tests and paid sixty dollars for each test, plus office call charges and the fertility pills which cost her at least twenty dollars a month. She took the fertility pills for a year, then her husband lost his job and they no longer could afford the expense of the doctors, tests and pills. Ann was also concerned about the way her body was reacting; she called it a weird feeling with slowed-down body functions. A friend told her about vitamin E and herbs and she decided to try them. She took high amounts of vitamin E, kelp and a B-complex vitamin. She was on this program for about three months and became pregnant. She said she would never take another fertility pill.

Julie also decided to change to vitamin E from the fertility pill. She had been through numerous tests, office calls and pills. She was unhappy about the way the pills made her feel emotionally. She suffered extreme mood changes. She stopped taking the pill and started on vitamin E, A, C, multiple vitamins, skullcap and red raspberry. Within five months she became pregnant.

These are not unusual cases. Vitamin E has helped hundreds of childless couples. Not only will it help in fertility but is a natural way to fight disease with nutrition. It is not a drug, but an essential food for the human body.

FACTS AT A GLANCE

- Cleanse the body of toxins through diet and supplements.
- Avoiding toxic chemicals greatly decreases the potential for fertility problems.
- Identifying your "fertile period" could help in targeting the optimal time window in which to attempt conceiving.
- Take supplements such as damiana, vitamin E and false unicorn to enhance fertility.
- Have the man examine any risk factors in his lifestyle that would contribute to decreased sperm production.

Miscellaneous Issues

SUGAR

It's sweet, fluffy, and ubiquitous — that solace for sorrow and panacea for pain called sugar. This seemingly harmless substance is actually an addicting drug, and it tears down the human body relatively quickly. Health author William Dufty, in his book *Sugar Blues*, states: "Hapless [sugar] addicts have been medically mistreated over the years with everything from morphine to tranquilizers, from brain surgery to burnings at the stake. How did a great civilization ever slide into such a stupefying bind?"

The intake of white, refined sugar is perhaps responsible for more human ills — both physical and psychological — than the average person ever imagined. It has been linked to diseases such as cancer and diabetes, but has also been linked to PMS, depression, heart problems, tooth decay, digestive disturbances and many other ailments.

Sugar is an empty carbohydrate that robs the body of nutrients such as calcium, magnesium, chromium, zinc, vitamin C and B-vitamins. Calcium and magnesium are responsible for strong bones and nervous system. Excessive, prolonged sugar intake can contribute to weak bones (including osteoporosis) and nervous disorders. It is hard to cope with stress when calcium, and magnesium, as well as B-vitamin reserves are low.

The adrenal glands depend upon good nutrition to function properly, and sugar can rob them of the necessary nutrients. These glands, which produce hormones in response to stress, can become "tired" when overworked. The adrenal glands help balance blood sugar levels, and when blood sugar levels are low (hypoglycemia), fatigue can result.

Chromium is the major nutrient responsible for a healthy pancreas. When the pancreas is not functioning properly, diabetes can result.

Zinc and vitamin C are major nutrients which help the body heal and repair tissues. They are also directly involved in keeping the body's immune system in good shape. If they are destroyed by sugar, a person is more susceptible to illness and chronic disease.

B-vitamins help keep a person's mental health balanced. When these nutrients are destroyed, mental illness can result. This problem can be manifested early as depression and mood swings. However, more severe symptoms can result. Schizophrenia has been linked to severe B-vitamin depletion. B-vitamins are responsible for keeping estrogen levels balanced in the body. When a woman produces excess estrogen that her body does not metabolize with the help of proper nutrients to nourish the liver, she can experience many premenstrual disorders, including painful cramps, water retention and moodiness. In extreme cases, suicidal thoughts are not uncommon.

The liver can become congested and sick from a diet rich in sugar. Because the liver is directly responsible for filtering toxins, including excessive estrogen, from the body, the immune system can go haywire and not perform its job when the a person eats a lot of sugar. This makes one more susceptible to illness, including chronic disease such as cancer.

The menstrual cycle gives a woman's body the opportunity to detoxify wastes every month, being partly a cleansing process. It is estimated that if she consumes a nutritious diet and stays away from junk foods, that the cycle could be shortened to 2-3 days.

Nancy Appleton, Ph.D., explains in her very informative book, *Lick the Sugar Habit:* "In addition to throwing off the body's homeostasis, excess sugar may result in a number of other significant consequences. Using documentation from a variety of medical journals and other scientific publications, I have summed up the consequences of a body out of homeostasis due to eating excess sugar." The following is the list Appleton came up with:

- *Sugar can suppress the immune system* (A. Sanchez, et al. "Role of Sugars in Human Neutrophilic Phagocytosis." *American Journal of Clinical Nutrition,* November 1973, pp. 1180-1184).
- *Sugar can upset the body's mineral balance* (F. Couizy, C. Keen, M.E. Gershwin, and F.P. Mareschi. "Nutritional Implications of the Interaction Between Minerals." *Progressive Food and Nutrition Science* 17, 1933, pp. 65-87).
- *Sugar can produce a significant rise in triglycerides* (S. Scanto, and John

Yudkin. "The Effect of Dietary Sucrose on Blood Lipids, Serum Insulin, Platelet Adhesiveness and Body Weight in Human Volunteers." *Postgraduate Medicine Journal* 45, 1969, pp. 602-607).

- *Sugar contributes to a weakened defense against bacterial infection* (W. Ringsdorf, E. Cheraskin, and R. Ramsay. "Sucrose Neutrophilic Phagocytosis and Resistance to Disease." *Dental Survey* 52, No. 12, 1976, pp. 46-48).
- *Sugar can cause kidney damage* (J. Yudkin, S. Kang, and K. Bruckdorfer. "Effects of High Dietary Sugar." *British Journal of Medicine* 281, November 22, 1980, p. 1396).
- *Sugar can reduce helpful high density lipoproteins* (HDLs) (Ibid).
- *Sugar can promote an elevation of harmful low density lipoproteins* (LDLs). (R. Pamplona, M.J. Bellmunt, M. Portero, and J. Prat. "Mechanisms of Glycation in Atherogenesis." *Medical Hypothesis* 40, 1990, pp. 174-181).
- *Sugar may lead to chromium deficiency* (A. Kozlovsky, et al. "Effects of Diets High in Simple Sugars on Urinary Chromium Losses." *Metabolism* 35, June 1986, pp. 515-518).
- *Sugar interferes with absorption of calcium and magnesium* (J. Lemann. "Evidence That Glucose Ingestion Inhibits Net Renal Tubular Reabsorption of Calcium and Magnesium." *Journal of Clinical Nutrition* 70, 1967, pp. 236-245).
- *Sugar can cause colon cancer, with an increased risk in women* (R.M. Bostick, J.d. Potter, L.H. Kushi, et al. "Sugar, Meat, and Fat Intake, and Non-dietary Risk Factors for Colon Cancer Incidence in Iowa Women." *Cancer Causes and Controls* 5, 1994, pp. 38-52).

Besides the above problems, sugar also sabotages the efforts of every person who has ever tried to lose weight. Sugar converts to fat in the body, and it can be stored all over, especially in places where you do not want it! In addition, excessive fat causes the body to produce excessive estrogen, which increases the chances for breast, uterine and ovarian cancer. A low-sugar, high-fiber diet helps the body to minimize the chances for cancer.

White refined sugar is hidden in many foods including ketchup, canned foods, frozen foods, etc. Read labels! It can come disguised as high fructose corn syrup or sucrose. Neither do you want to ingest commercial sugar substitutes, such as aspartame (NutraSweet®). This substance has been linked to seizures, migraine headaches, and even more important ailments.

Dr. H.J. Roberts has written an excellent book on the dangers of aspartame called *Aspartame (NutraSweet®) — Is it Safe?* He states that a type of brain tumor known as a primary lymphoma of the brain, may be associated with NutraSweet®. This tumor has a high mortality rate, meaning that often people who come down with it do not live very long.

It is said that "looks can be deceiving." You would think that something that is white and sweet would be pure and good. Not in the case of sugar!

Mass-Market Refining

Mass market refining is concerned with getting the job done as quickly and cheaply as possible. Petroleum (petrochemical) solvents are used to yield the oils from the grain seeds used in the hundreds of different food items. Some companies also utilize caustic soda and acid-based clays during the refining and bleaching phases of refining. Following the bleaching stage, harmful substances known as peroxides may form in the oils, as a result of the oxidation and breaking down process. Free radicals are often found in peroxidized oils. When the oils are finally heated to high temperatures in the final refining stage, most of the nutrients that may have escaped annihilation are finally destroyed.

What are Free Radicals?

Technically, a free radical is an element or molecule with an unpaired electron. If not limited and controlled, they can damage the body's cells and accelerate the processes of disease and aging. Certain enzymes and nutrients known as "antioxidants" will scavenge for free radicals and neutralize them, preventing them from harming the body. Thus, they are known as "free radical scavengers." These nutrients include vitamins C and E, and beta carotene (provitamin A), grape seed extract, selenium and zinc, and the enzymes glutathione peroxidase and superoxide dismutase (SOD). There are a host of others, including herbs, which are too numerous to mention. Some signs of free radical damage to the body may include premature aging, brown (liver) spots on the skin, cancer, arthritis and cross-linking (causing wrinkles).

Bibliography and Recommended Reading

In addition to the references already mentioned throughout the book, the following are also excellent sources of information:

Appleton, Nancy, Ph.D.
Lick the Sugar Habit, 1996
Healthy Bones, Avery Publishing Group

Breggin, Peter R., M.D.
Toxic Psychiatry, 1991
St. Martin's Press, New York, N.Y.

Brown, Donald J., N.D.
Herbal Prescriptions for Better Health, 1996..
Prima Publishing, Rocklin, CA.

Cichoke, Anthony J., D.C.
Enzymes and Enzyme Therapy
Keats Publishing, Inc.

Cameron, Myra
Lifetime Encyclopedia of Natural Remedies, 1993.
Parker Publishing Co., Inc.
West Nyack, N.Y.

Cousens, Gabriel, M.D.
Conscious Eating, 1992
Vision Books International
Santa Rosa, CA

Casdorph, H. Richard, Dr. and Walker, Mordon, Dr.
Toxic Metal Syndrome, 1995
Avery Publishing Group
Garden City Park, N.J.

Elkins, Rita, M.A.
The Complete Home Health Advisor, 1994.
Depression and Natural Medicine, 1995.
The Complete Fiber Fact Book, 1996.
Woodland Health Books, Pleasant Grove, Utah

Gladstar, Rosemary
Herbal Healing for Women, 1993.
Fireside, New York, N.Y.

Harrison, Lewis
Helping Yourself with Natural Healing, 1988.
Prentice Hall
Englewood Cliffs, N.J.

Jensen, Bernard, D.C., N.D.
Iridology, The Science and Practice of the Healing Arts, 1982
Bernard Jensen, Publisher.
Escondido, CA.
Beyond Basic Health, 1988.
Avery Publishing Group.

Kellogg, John Harvey, M.D.
Colon Hygiene, 1916.
Good Health Publishing Co.
Battle Creek, Michigan.

Koch, Carolee Bateson, D.C., N.D.
Allergies: Disease in Disguise, 1994.
Alive Books
Burnaby, B.C., Canada

Leuna, Albert Y. and Foster, Steven.
Encyclopedia of Common Natural Ingredients Used in Food, Drug and Cosmetics, Second Edition: 1996
John Wiley and Sons, Inc.

Lane, Sir W. Arbuthnot, M.D.
The Prevention of the Diseases Peculiar to Civilization
Reissued, 1981 by Foundation for Alternative Cancer Therapies, Ltd.
New York, N.Y.

Ley, Beth M.
Natural Healing Handbook, 1990.
Christopher Lawrence Communications
United States of America

Lark, Susan M., M.D.
Fibroid Tumors and Endometriosis, 1993.
Westchester Publishing Co.
Los Altos, CA.

Lin, David J.
Free Radicals and Disease Prevention, 1993.
Keats Publishing, Inc.
New Cameron, Connecticut

LePore, Donald, N.D.
The Ultimate Healing System
Woodland Health Books

Murray, Michael, N.D. and Pizzorno, Joseph, N.D.
Encyclopedia of Natural Medicine, 1991.
Primar Publishing
Rocklin, CA.

Murray, Michael T., N.D.
The Healing Power of Foods, 1993.
Stress, Anxiety, and Insomnia, 1995.
Prima Publishing
Rocklin, CA.

Monte, Tom and Editors of East West Natural Health
World Medicine, 1993.
The Putnam Publishing Group.
New York, N.Y.

Rogers, Sherry A., M.D.
Wellness Against All Odds, 1994.
Prestige Publishing
Syracuse, N.Y.

Rona, Zoltan, M.D., MSc.
Return to the Joy of Health, 1995.
Alive Books
Burnaby B.C. Canada

Sharon, Michael Dr.
Complete Nutrition, 1989.
Prion
London, England

Scott, Julian and Susan.
Natural Medicine for Women, 1991.
Gaia Books
New York, N.Y.

Stein, Diane
The Natural Remedy Book for Women, 1992.
The Crossing Press.

Santillo, Humbart "Smokey", N.D.
Intuitive Eating, 1993.
Food Enzymes, The Missing Link to Radiant Health, 1987.
Hohm Press,
Prescott, AZ.

Tenney, Louise, M.H.,
Today's Herbal Health, 1980, Revised 1992.
Today's Healthy Eating, 1986.
Modern-Day Plagues, 1987. Revised 1994.
Health Handbook, 1987. Revised 1996.
Nutritional Guide, 1994.
The Encyclopedia of Natural Remedies, 1995.
Today's Herbal Health for Children, 1996.
Woodland Publishing, Inc.
Pleasant Grove, Utah

Weil, Andrew, M.D. and Rosen, Winifred.
Chocolate to Morphine, 1983.
Houghton Mifflin Co.
Boston, Massachusetts

Weinberger, Stanley
Healing Within, 1988.
Desktop Publishing
Mill Valley, CA.

Index

acne 93,124,190,193
acidophilus 13,20,24,32,43,46,48,52,58, 70,116,128,133,207
addictions 142–47
adrenal glands 15,24,89,104–10,150,211 231
alcohol 17,19,27,33,39,54,104,114,141,164,168,199,224
alfalfa 13,64,80,94,106,150,172,178,189,226
aloe vera 16,25,28,46,49,166
allergies 33,42–43,63,92,125–29,148,170
anemia 44,68,75–78,192,203
anorexia 11
antioxidants 18,21,24,36,42,50,234
anxiety 147–51
appestat 14,117
arthritis 174–79
autointoxication 32–35,123,148,156,158–159
balding 193
barberry 138,150
barley 35,100,138,224
bayberry 84,148
bile 14,43,110,168
black cohosh 94,166,198,214,220
black currant 13,28,43,128,146,216
black walnut 27,76,84,110,114,139
bladder, infections of 54–59
blessed thistle 171,196,220
blue-green algae 16,21,35,50,65,78,113,128,136,146,159,163,195
blue vervain 127,161
bone loss 186–90

borage 26,43,69,124,146,152,163,177,218
breast, cancer of 211
bronchitis 62–65
buchu 57–58
buckthorn bark 36,70
burdock 16,29,43,77,139,146,178,199,207
butcher's broom 65,81
calcium 36,12,21,36,57,78,84,92,94,106,124,129,146,178,
    182–190,222, 229
calories 112–115,222
cancer 121–25
Candida albicans 20,112,130–134,166,214
candidiasis (see Candida albicans)
capsicum 28,46,81,139
carpal tunnel syndrome 183–85
cascara sagrada 84,139,146,162,
catnip 21,138
cat's claw 28,36,44,50,94,101,110,124,133,139,178,185,199,
    207,215
cayenne 76,81,150,176
cellulite 116–17
chamomile 29,94,154,166
chemical imbalances 151–55
chlorophyll 13,15,18,24,35,46,59,65,107,117,128,136,146,195,207
chocolate 93,105,142,144,187
cholesterol 14,82,98,116,217,219,222–223
chronic fatigue syndrome 134–36
circulatory system 73
coffee 27,57,77,121,143,145,148
colds 22,36,63,65–67,71,200
colon 18,23,25,31–52,60,74,104,117,125,146,150,158–160,193,
    194
comfrey 29,102,139,189
constipation 16,19,28,33–41,48,56,62,92,108,126,224
cough 65–70,121,126
cramps, muscle 99,108,126

cranberries 56
Crohn's Disease 44–47
cysts 95–99
dandelion (root) 29,102,125,149,215,225
depression 11,33,69,92–94,111,143,155–159,200,202
diabetes 99–102,108,231
diarrhea 37,51,104,137
digestive system 9
diverticulitis 47–50
dong quai 71,94,200,215,223
drugs 19,22,24,54,67,113,137,151,157,160,220,224
dulse 80,108
ear problems 165–68
achinacea 28,58,98,206
emphysema 62–5
endometriosis 96,213,226
enema 32,56,138
ephedra 115
Epstein Barr virus 134–36
essential fatty acids 11,25,28,50,71,82,124,136,148,150,163,178,
    195,215–216
estrogen 14,24,36,92–98,116–121,158,186–188,203,209–13
evening primrose (see essential fatty acids) 94,216
exercise 14,32–38,52,64–65,70,83,100,110–113,116,135–136,
    153,161, 176,184,188,222
false unicorn 171,200
fatigue 22,33,38,75,90,122,126,132–136,158,168,174,208
fats 14,51,84,99,113–117,123,131,180,215–18
fennel 150,162
fertility 96,198,200,203,212,220,227–30
fever 14,48,65–72,122,137,170,174,202
fiber 14–50,82,100,122,132,159,204–206,210,218
fibrocitis 180–83
fibromyalgia 179–80
fingernails 192–96
flaxseed (see essential fatty acids) 133

food enzymes 28
free radicals 104,109,124,153,234
gallbladder 13–16,58
garlic 58,70,98,124,133,139
gentian (root) 77,127
germanium 13,45,63,107,117,124,133,136
ginger 29,128,132,46,150,199
ginkgo 13,81,98,150,154,158,168,185
ginseng 90,159,168,172
glandular system 83
goldenseal 13,18,28,46,58,102,106,115,167
gotu kola 81,98,150,154,168
guar gum 29
hair 192–96
   gray 186
hawthorn 81,185
headache 19,29,69,92,158,181,223
   migraine 169–72
hemorrhoids 39,82,84,126,198
hiatal hernia 16–19
H. pylori 25
hops 13,151,182
ho-shou-wu 71
hydrangea 58
hydrochloric acid 18–25,35,42,65,146
hypoglycemia 103–7
hypothyroidism 107
hysterectomy 46,213,220
immune system 22,40,58,81,92,98–101,119–140,175,197,200,206,
   226
indigestion 19–21,39,122,143,198,224
inflammatory bowel disease 44
insomnia 39,92,168,172
insulin 88,90,99–103
integumentary system 191
intestinal system 31–52,71,94,127,133,139,158,199,202,215

Irish moss 109,127
irritable bowel syndrome 50–2
joints 21,67,89,126,134,137,161,174–182,208
juniper berries 58,102
kelp 13,98,108,110,115,150,162,175,182,189,225
kidneys 32,53-59,99,123,170,199,205
  infections of 54–59
lady's slipper 155
Lane, Arbuthnot 38
leaky gut syndrome 21–24
Lecithin 15
licorice 18,28,45,106,150,168,201
lobelia (see nervine herbs)
lupus 136–39
lymphatic system 73
magnesium 36,59,78,94,106,124,129,150,178,182,188,205,228
marshmallow 64
Menniere's Syndrome (see tinnitus)
menopause 94,147,190,201,212,214,220–24,227
milk thistle 29,136,151,201,206
mononucleosis 136
mullein 65,84
muscle disorders 179–83
myrrh 29,127
nausea 19,22,26,51,70,126,164,202–204,221
nervine herbs 47,65,90,139,154,163
nervous system 141
obesity 110–16
Omega-3 fatty acids 177,218
Oregon grape 35,43,139
osteoporosis 186–90
ovaries, cancer of 211
pancreas 26,89,90,99–103,231
panic attacks 147–151
papaya 49
parasites 22,25,35,44–52,101,110,126,138–139,176,199

parsley 58,162,214
passion flower (see nervine herbs)
pau d'arco 123,133,139,203
periodontal disease 186
peach bark 36,150
pineal gland 90
pituitary gland 90
plant digestive enzyme 12,24,42,50,64
plantain 65
pregnancy 33,37,54,58,83,110,198,200,202,219,224–227
premenstrual syndrome (PMS) 91–95,164,200,215,231
prickly ash bark 36,150
psyllium husk 49
pumpkin seed 34,127
red clover 47,125,202
red respberry 29,198,202
rejuvelac 27
respiratory system 61
rose hips 65,89
rosemary 114
rhubarb root 150
St. John's wort (see nervine herbs) 172,202
salt 14,17,80,106,114,139,177,187
sarsaparilla 115,202
selenium 24,84,124,171,229
senna 70
silicon breast implants 204–7
skin 11,19,31–35,55,68,74,79,93,99,117,121,123,136,192–96
skullcap (see nervine herbs)
slippery elm 46,85
smoking 62
Staphlycoccus aureus 205
stress 10,17,19,26,27,32,44,48,50,80,88,92,106,111,134,147–50,
    172,183,195,217,228
structural system 173
sugar 17,33,47,49,77,93,99–107,122,130–142,161,186,230–234

tampons 204–7
tea 29,70
thyme 65
thymus gland 89
thyroid gland 90
tinnitus 164–168,200
tobacco 39,41,101,139,142–144,194
toxic shock syndrome 204–7
tumors 95–9
ulcers 25–9
urinary system 53–59,186,233
urine 53–59,122,208
uterus 51,92–94,198–99,202
    cancer of 211
uva ursi 59,102
valerian root (see nervine herbs)
vision 59,102
Vitamin A 24,49,71,84,93,101,106,124,133,195,229
Vitamin B 124,165,185
    B-complex 13,15,43,50,64,78,93,101,106,117,136,145,154,171,
    207,227
Vitamin C 15,24,36,64,78,84,94,117,133,150,185,226
Vitamin D 84,124,189,219,226
Vitamin E 15,43,71,84,101,117,133,182,226,229–230
Vitamin K 24,226
vomiting 14,22,48,126,137,164,169,221
watercress 18,77,97,110
wheatgrass 30,46,65,71,123,145,228
white willow (see nervine herbs)
wild yam 95,172,203,215,223
wood betony (see nervine herbs)
yellow dock 47,77,151,192,202,226
zinc (see antioxidants) 12,78,84,101,171,185,189,226,229